A SECOND CHICKEN SOUP FOR THE WOMAN'S SOUL

101 *More* Stories
to Open the Hearts and
Rekindle the Spirits of Women

Jack Canfield
Mark Victor Hansen
Jennifer Read Hawthorne
Marci Shimoff

Vermilion
LONDON

9 10

Published in 2004 by Vermilion, an imprint of Ebury Publishing
First published in the USA by Health Communications, Inc. in 1998

Ebury Publishing is a Random House Group company

The Random House Group Limited Reg. No. 954009

Addresses for companies within the Random House Group
can be found at: www.randomhouse.co.uk

A CIP catalogue record for this book is available from the British Library

The Random House Group Limited supports The Forest Stewardship
Council (FSC®), the leading international forest certification organisation.
Our books carrying the FSC label are printed on FSC® certified paper. FSC is
the only forest certification scheme endorsed by the leading environmental
organisations, including Greenpeace. Our paper procurement policy can be
found at www.randomhouse.co.uk/environment

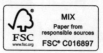

Printed and bound by
CPI Group (UK) Ltd, Croydon, CR0 4YY

ISBN 9780091899998

Copies are available at special rates for bulk orders. Contact the sales
development team on 020 7840 8487 for more information.

To buy books by your favourite authors and register for offers, visit
www.randomhouse.co.uk

With gratitude,
we dedicate this book to
Mother Teresa
and to all women
who answer the call to
share their hearts
and love.

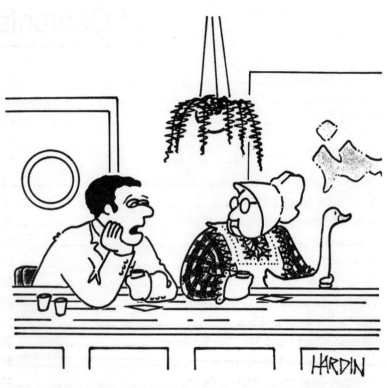

"You look like a lady with a story to tell."

Contents

2. ON ATTITUDE

3. LIVE YOUR DREAMS

4. ON MARRIAGE

8. SPECIAL MOMENTS

9. MIRACLES

10. ACROSS THE GENERATIONS

Acknowledgments

A Second Chicken Soup for the Woman's Soul has taken more than a year to write, compile and edit. It has been a true labor of love for all of us. One of the greatest joys of creating this book was working with people who gave this project not just their time and attention, but their hearts and souls as well. We would like to thank the following people for their dedication and contributions, without which this book could not have been created:

Our families, who have given us love and support throughout this project, and have been chicken soup for *our* souls!

Dan Hawthorne, whose unconditional acceptance, enthusiasm for our work and great sense of humor always keep us going. Thank you for being one of our biggest fans.

Amy and William Hawthorne, for sharing their youthful perspective and being part of our cheering section.

Maureen H. Read, for always being there for us.

Louise and Marcus Shimoff, who are always thinking of us and providing love and support on every level.

Georgia Noble, for her love and her gracious support while we worked on this project.

Christopher Noble Canfield, for sharing his innocence, his art, his singing, his acting, his great hugs and his irre-pressible love for life with us.

Patty Hansen, and Elisabeth and Melanie Hansen, for once again sharing and lovingly supporting us in the process of creating yet another book.

Patty Aubery, the glue that holds everything together at the central *Chicken Soup for the Soul* office. Your heart, your clarity and your dedication are a constant inspiration, and we always appreciate how much we can count on you.

Beverly Merson, for putting her heart and soul into this project. We are grateful for your extraordinary talents in researching and creative problem-solving, and for your great dedication to this book. We thank you from the bottom of our hearts.

Elinor Hall, who did an extraordinary job in helping us read and research stories for this book. We deeply appreciate your support, your love and your friendship.

Carol Kline, for her wonderful contributions in researching, writing and editing stories for this book. Carol, you are a brilliant writer and we are grateful for your talent and your never-ending friendship.

Cynthia Knowlton and Sue Penberthy, for their devoted support and care of Jennifer's and Marci's respective lives. Thank you for keeping us sane. We couldn't have done this without both of you.

Sharon Linnéa, Erica Orloff and Wendy Miles, for their marvelous job of editing numerous stories. Your editor's touch captured the essence of *Chicken Soup*.

Joanne Cox, for an outstanding job typing and preparing our initial manuscripts. Thank you for your great attention to detail and your loyalty to this project.

Craig Herndon, our information management hero, for assisting with the preparation of the initial manuscript.

Suzanne Thomas Lawlor, for her excellent contributions in researching and reading hundreds of story submissions.

Jeanette Lisefski, for keeping parts of our office impeccably on track.

Peter Vegso and Gary Seidler at Health Communications, Inc., our publishers extraordinaire, for their vision and their commitment to bringing *Chicken Soup for the Soul* to the world.

Heather McNamara, senior editor for the *Chicken Soup for the Soul* series, for working with us throughout the process of compiling this book, and for preparing and editing our final manuscript. You are a pro and a joy to work with!

Nancy Mitchell, for managing the ever-challenging process of obtaining permissions for the stories used in this book—and somehow staying sane through it all. Thanks for your invaluable help.

Leslie Forbes, who was always there when we needed her and always had a smile on her face and love in her heart.

Veronica Romero and Robin Yerian, for working in Jack's office to make sure everything ran smoothly during the production of this book.

Rosalie Miller, who kept all of the communication flowing efficiently throughout this project. Your smiling face and never-ending encouragement have lightened our hearts.

Teresa Esparza, who brilliantly coordinated all of Jack's speaking, travel, and radio and television appearances during this time.

Kimberly Kirberger, for her ongoing support in all areas.

Larry and Linda Price, who, in addition to keeping Jack's Foundation for Self-Esteem operating smoothly, continue to administrate the Soup Kitchens for the Soul project, which distributes thousands of *Chicken Soup for the Soul* books free each year to prisoners, halfway houses, homeless shelters, battered women's shelters and inner city schools.

John and Shannon Tullius, John Saul, Mike Sacks, Bud Gardner, Dan Poynter, Bryce Courtney, Terry Brooks and all our other friends at the Maui Writers Conference and Retreat who inspire and encourage us every year.

Christine Belleris, Matthew Diener, Lisa Drucker and Allison Janse, our editors at Health Communications, for their generous efforts in bringing this book to its high state of excellence.

Randee Goldsmith, *Chicken Soup for the Soul* manager at Health Communications, for her masterful coordination and support of all the *Chicken Soup* projects.

Terry Burke, Irene Xanthos, Jane Barone, Lori Golden, Kelly Johnson Maragni, Karen Baliff Ornstein and Yvonne zum Tobel, the people at Health Communications, responsible for selling and marketing the *Chicken Soup* books.

Kim Weiss, Larry Getlen and Ronni O'Brien at Health Communications, for their publicity and marketing efforts.

Andrea Perrine Brower at Health Communications, for working with us so patiently and cooperatively on the cover design of this book.

Robbin O'Neill, and George and Felicity Foster, for their artistic input and invaluable ideas on cover design.

Rochelle Pennington, for assisting us with quotes.

Sandra McCormick Hill and Lynn Ramage at *Reader's Digest* and Maria Porzio at Economics Press, who generously go out of their way to help us.

Jim Rubis and the Fairfield (Iowa) Public Library, and Tony Kainauskas, Arnie Wolfson and Shirley Norway at 21st Century Bookstore, for their outstanding research assistance.

Fairfield Printing, especially Stephanie Harward and

Cindy Sharp, for their enthusiastic support of our work.

Tom Simmons and Sherry Johnson at the Fairfield Post Office, for assistance above and beyond the call of duty.

Jerry Teplitz, for his inventive approach to testing manuscript and cover design.

John Reiner, who nourished our bodies and souls with his exquisite food during the final weeks of the project.

Robert Kenyon, for always being there with love, humor and support.

Debra Poneman, for her inspiration.

Terry Johnson and Bill Levacy, for their astute guidance on aspects of this project.

M., for the gifts of wisdom and knowledge.

Ann Blanchard, for her strength, clarity and loving guidance on this project.

The following people, who supported and encouraged us during this project: Ron Hall, Amsheva Miller, Birgitte Necessary, Paul and Susan Shimoff, and Lynda Valles.

We extend our gratitude to the following people, who completed the monumental task of reading the preliminary manuscript of this book, helped us make the final selections, and made invaluable comments on how to improve the book: Christine Belleris, Carolyn Burch, Diana Chapman, Linda DeGraaff, Lisa Drucker, Leslie Forbes, Mary Gagnon, Randee Goldsmith, Elinor Hall, Amy Hawthorne, Carol Jackson, Allison Janse, Carol Kline, Jeanette Lisefski, Kathy Karocki, Cynthia Knowlton, Robin Kotok, Ariane Luckey, Barbara McLoughlin, Karen McLoughlin, Heather McNamara, Barbara McQuaide, Beverly Merson, Holly Moore, Sandra Moradi, Sue Penberthy, Maureen H. Read, Wendy Read, Karen Rosenstein, Heather Sanders, Marcus and Louise Shimoff, Belinda Stroup, and Lynda Valles.

We also thank the following people, who took the time to spread the word about this book and helped us

xviii ACKNOWLEDGMENTS

network with other writers: Terry Marotta, Marsha Arons, Jean Ravenscroft, Rob Spiegel, Eddy Hall, Marilyn Strube, Melanie Hemry, Maxine Holder, Marlene Bagnull, Bob Lightman, Carol Zetterberger, Pam Gordon, Ray Newton, Marion Bond West, John Fuhrman, Robyn Weaver, Susan Osborne, Meera Lester, Reg A. Forder, Elaine Colvin Wright, Elizabeth Klungness, Anita Gilbert and Marden Burr Mitchel.

We deeply appreciate all the *Chicken Soup for the Soul* coauthors, who make it a joy to be part of this *Chicken Soup* family: Patty Aubery, Marty Becker, Ron Camacho, Irene Dunlap, Patty Hansen, Kimberly Kirberger, Tim Clauss, Carol Kline, Hanoch McCarty, Meladee McCarty, Nancy Mitchell, Maida Rogerson, Martin Rutte, Barry Spilchuk and Diana von Welanetz Wentworth.

We also wish to acknowledge the hundreds of people who sent us stories, poems and quotes for possible inclusion in *A Second Chicken Soup for the Woman's Soul.* While we were not able to use everything you sent in, we were deeply touched by your heartfelt intention to share yourselves and your stories with our readers and us. Many of these may be used in future volumes of *Chicken Soup for the Soul.* Thank you!

Because of the size of this project, we may have left out the names of some people who helped us along the way. If so, we are sorry—please know that we really do appreciate all of you very deeply.

We are truly grateful for the many hands and hearts that have made this book possible. We love you all!

Introduction

Welcome to *A Second Chicken Soup for the Woman's Soul: 101 More Stories to Open the Hearts and Rekindle the Spirits of Women*.

Since the first *Chicken Soup for the Woman's Soul* came out, we have been overwhelmed by the response from readers around the world. The book has been at the top of every major bestseller's list in the United States, and it continues to be read by millions.

But what has moved us most is the feedback about how the stories have touched the lives of women around the world. Our goal in writing that book was to open the hearts and touch the souls of women everywhere. Apparently, that happened.

In fact, many readers told us that these stories are like potato chips—once you start, you can't read just one. The letters and comments we have received have been so moving and inspiring that we wanted to share a few with you.

From the Bahamas: "It was just absolutely one of the best books I have read for a long time. When I was about halfway into the book, I deliberately slowed down because I did not want the beautiful stories to end."

From New Zealand: ". . . after reading this book, I can honestly say that I say more thank-yous, and as I climb into a warm bed at night, I count my blessings."

From Michigan: "The stories made me cry—not out of sadness but out of joy. I said to myself, 'Who are these women and how come I don't know them? They are so much like me, sometimes struggling but with an amazing sense of self.' I found myself then saying, 'I do know them. *I am them.*'"

From California: "I suffer from depression. I've never wanted to take anti-depressants due to their side effects. Your books work as my medication. As long as I am able to read at least a story or two a day, I feel okay. Being a single mom, life is hard enough, but your books give me what I need to make it a little easier."

We are often asked why the *Chicken Soup for the Soul* books have become such a phenomenon. From our experience, people seem to be soul-starved. With all the bad news that we hear all day long, people are relieved to hear these true stories of hope, courage, love and inspiration. They nourish the soul.

Mother Teresa has said:

> *The greatest disease in the West today is not TB or leprosy; it is being unwanted, unloved and uncared for. We can cure physical diseases with medicine, but the only cure for loneliness, despair and hopelessness is love. There are many in the world who are dying for a piece of bread, but there are many more dying for a little love. The poverty in the West is a different kind of poverty—it is not only a poverty of loneliness but also of spirituality. There's a hunger for love. . . .*

The stories in *A Second Chicken Soup for the Woman's Soul* are about ordinary people doing extraordinary things. We are happy to celebrate the good in people and we hope that this "soup" helps satisfy, even in some small way, the hunger for love in the world.

Share with Us

We would love to hear your reactions to the stories in this book. Please let us know what your favorite stories were and how they affected you.

We also invite you to send us stories you would like to see published in future editions of *Chicken Soup for the Woman's Soul.* You can send us either stories you have written or stories written by others that you have liked.

Send your submissions to:

Chicken Soup for the Woman's Soul
P.O. Box 1959, Dept. WS2
Fairfield, IA 52556
e-mail: *chickensoup@lisco.com*
phone: 800-211-5948
fax: 515-472-7288

You can also access e-mail or find a current list of planned books at the *Chicken Soup for the Soul* site at *www.chickensoup.com.* Find out about our Internet service at *www.clubchickensoup.com.*

We hope you enjoy reading this book as much as we enjoyed compiling, editing and writing it.

DENNIS THE MENACE

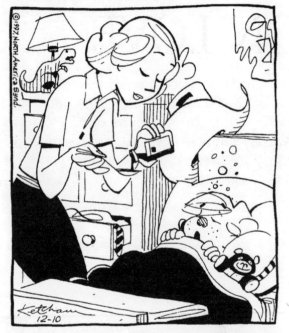

"What ever happened to Chicken Soup?"

1

ON LOVE

Nobody has ever measured, not even poets, how much the heart can hold.

Zelda Fitzgerald

The Wallet

As I walked home one freezing day, I stumbled on a wallet someone had lost in the street. I picked it up and looked inside to find some identification so I could call the owner. But the wallet contained only three dollars and a crumpled letter that looked as if it had been in there for years.

The envelope was worn and the only thing that was legible on it was the return address. I started to open the letter, hoping to find some clue. Then I saw the dateline—1924. The letter had been written almost sixty years earlier.

It was written in a beautiful feminine handwriting, on powder-blue stationery with a little flower in the left-hand corner. It was a "Dear John" letter that told the recipient, whose name appeared to be Michael, that the writer could not see him any more because her mother forbade it. Even so, she wrote that she would always love him. It was signed Hannah.

It was a beautiful letter, but there was no way, except for the name Michael, to identify the owner. Maybe if I called information, the operator could find a phone listing for the address on the envelope.

"Operator," I began, "this is an unusual request. I'm trying to find the owner of a wallet that I found. Is there any way you can tell me if there is a phone number for an address that was on an envelope in the wallet?"

She suggested I speak with her supervisor, who hesitated for a moment, then said, "Well, there is a phone listing at that address, but I can't give you the number." She said as a courtesy, she would call that number, explain my story and ask whoever answered if the person wanted her to connect me. I waited a few minutes and then the supervisor was back on the line. "I have a party who will speak with you."

I asked the woman on the other end of the line if she knew anyone by the name of Hannah. She gasped. "Oh! We bought this house from a family who had a daughter named Hannah. But that was thirty years ago!"

"Would you know where that family could be located now?" I asked.

"I remember that Hannah had to place her mother in a nursing home some years ago," the woman said. "Maybe if you got in touch with them, they might be able to track down the daughter."

She gave me the name of the nursing home, and I called the number. The woman on the phone told me the old lady had passed away some years ago, but the nursing home did have a phone number for where the daughter might be living.

I thanked the person at the nursing home and phoned the number she gave me. The woman who answered explained that Hannah herself was now living in a nursing home.

This whole thing is stupid, I thought to myself. *Why am I making such a big deal over finding the owner of a wallet that has only three dollars and a letter that is almost sixty years old?*

Nevertheless, I called the nursing home in which Hannah was supposed to be living, and the man who answered the phone told me, "Yes, Hannah is staying with us."

Even though it was already 10 P.M., I asked if I could come by to see her. "Well," he said hesitatingly, "if you want to take a chance, she might be in the day room watching television."

I thanked him and drove over to the nursing home. The night nurse and a guard greeted me at the door. We went up to the third floor of the large building. In the day room, the nurse introduced me to Hannah. She was a sweet, silver-haired old-timer with a warm smile and a twinkle in her eye.

I told her about finding the wallet and showed her the letter. The second she saw the powder-blue envelope with that little flower on the left, she took a deep breath and said, "Young man, this letter was the last contact I ever had with Michael."

She looked away for a moment, deep in thought, and then said softly, "I loved him very much. But I was only sixteen at the time and my mother felt I was too young. Oh, he was so handsome. He looked like Sean Connery, the actor.

"Yes," she continued, "Michael Goldstein was a wonderful person. If you should find him, tell him I think of him often. And," she hesitated for a moment, almost biting her lip, "tell him I still love him. You know," she said, smiling as tears welled up in her eyes, "I never did marry. I guess no one ever matched up to Michael . . . "

I thanked Hannah and said good-bye. I took the elevator to the first floor and as I stood by the door, the guard there asked, "Was the old lady able to help you?"

I told him she had given me a lead. "At least I have a last name. But I think I'll let it go for a while. I spent almost the whole day trying to find the owner of this wallet."

I had taken out the wallet, which was a simple brown leather case with red lacing on the side. When the guard saw it, he said, "Hey, wait a minute! That's Mr. Goldstein's wallet. I'd know it anywhere with that bright red lacing. He's always losing that wallet. I must have found it in the halls at least three times."

"Who's Mr. Goldstein?" I asked, as my hand began to shake.

"He's one of the old-timers on the eighth floor. That's Mike Goldstein's wallet for sure. He must have lost it on one of his walks."

I thanked the guard and quickly ran back to the nurse's office. I told her what the guard had said. We went back to the elevator and got on. I prayed that Mr. Goldstein would be up.

On the eighth floor, the floor nurse said, "I think he's still in the day room. He likes to read at night. He's a darling old man."

We went to the only room that had any lights on, and there was a man reading a book. The nurse went over to him and asked if he had lost his wallet. Mr. Goldstein looked up with surprise, put his hand in his back pocket and said, "Oh, it *is* missing!"

"This kind gentleman found a wallet and we wondered if it could be yours."

I handed Mr. Goldstein the wallet, and the second he saw it, he smiled with relief and said, "Yes, that's it! It must have dropped out of my pocket this afternoon. I want to give you a reward."

"No, thank you," I said. "But I have to tell you something. I read the letter in the hope of finding out who owned the wallet."

The smile on his face suddenly disappeared. "You read that letter?"

"Not only did I read it, I think I know where Hannah is."

He suddenly grew pale. "Hannah? You know where she is? How is she? Is she still as pretty as she was? Please, please tell me," he begged.

"She's fine . . . just as pretty as when you knew her," I said softly.

The old man smiled with anticipation and asked, "Could you tell me where she is? I want to call her tomorrow." He grabbed my hand and said, "You know something, mister? I was so in love with that girl that when that letter came, my life literally ended. I never married. I guess I've always loved her."

"Michael," I said, "come with me."

We took the elevator down to the third floor. The hallways were darkened and only one or two little night lights lit our way to the day room, where Hannah was sitting alone, watching the television.

The nurse walked over to her.

"Hannah," she said softly, pointing to Michael, who was waiting with me in the doorway. "Do you know this man?"

She adjusted her glasses, looked for a moment, but didn't say a word.

Michael said softly, almost in a whisper, "Hannah, it's Michael. Do you remember me?"

She gasped. "Michael! I don't believe it! Michael! It's you! My Michael!"

He walked slowly toward her, and they embraced. The nurse and I left with tears streaming down our faces.

"See," I said. "See how the good Lord works! If it's meant to be, it will be."

About three weeks later, I got a call at my office from the nursing home. "Can you break away on Sunday to attend a wedding? Michael and Hannah are going to tie the knot!"

It was a beautiful wedding, with all the people at the nursing home dressed up to join in the celebration. Hannah wore a light beige dress and looked beautiful. Michael wore a dark blue suit and stood tall. They made me their best man.

The hospital gave them their own room, and if you ever wanted to see a seventy-six-year-old bride and a seventy-nine-year-old groom acting like two teenagers, you had to see this couple.

A perfect ending for a love affair that had lasted nearly sixty years.

Arnold Fine

A Gift for Robby

Little Robby, our neighbor's nephew, carefully spooned some of his water ration into a saucer and started for the door. How I hated this water rationing. We were forced to bathe without soap in the deep little pond we shared with Jessie, our cow. She was all we had now. Wells were dry, crops transformed to dust and blew away with our dreams, during the worst drought our small farming community had ever seen.

I held the screen open for Robby and watched, smiling, as he slowly sat on the steps. Dozens of bees circled his tousled brown curls in an angel's halo. He imitated their buzzing, which brought them to the saucer to sip the precious liquid.

His aunt's words echoed in my ears:

"I don't know what I was thinking when I took him in. Doctors say he wasn't hurt in the crash that killed my sister, but he can't talk. Oh, he makes noises all right, but they aren't human. He's in a world all his own, that boy, not like my children at all."

Why couldn't she see the wonderful gifts this four-year-old boy possessed? My heart ached for Robby. He had become the dearest part of our world, eagerly tending the garden with me and riding the tractor or pitching hay with my husband, Tom. He was blessed with a loving nature and a deep admiration for all living things, and I knew he could talk to animals.

We rejoiced in discoveries he joyfully shared with us. His inquisitive and often impish brown eyes mirrored an understanding of everything verbal. I longed to adopt him. His aunt had hinted often enough. We even called ourselves Mom and Dad to Robby, and before the drought had discussed adoption. But times were so bleak now that I couldn't approach the subject with Tom. The job he was forced to take in town to buy feed for Jessie and bare necessities for us had exacted its toll on his spirit.

Robby's aunt eagerly agreed to our request that he live with us for the summer. All his days were spent in our company anyway. I brushed away a tear, remembering how tiny and helpless he looked when she hastily put his hand in mine and gave me a rumpled brown paper bag. It contained two faded T-shirts we had bought him last year at the county fair and a hand-me-down pair of shorts. This and the clothes he wore were his only belongings, with the exception of one prized possession.

On a silken cord around his neck dangled a hand-carved whistle. Tom had made it for him in case he was ever lost or in danger. After all, he could not call out for help. He knew perfectly well that the whistle was not a toy. It was for emergencies only, and to blow on it would bring us both running. I had told him the story of the boy who cried wolf, and I knew he understood me.

I sighed as I dried and put away the last supper dish. Tom came into the kitchen and picked up the dishpan. Every ounce of recycled water was saved for a tiny vegetable garden Robby had planted beside the porch. He was so proud of it, we tried desperately to save it. But without rain soon, it too would be lost. Tom put the pan on the counter and turned to me.

"You know, honey," he started, "I've been thinking a lot about Robby lately."

My heart began to pound in anticipation, but before he could continue, a shrill blast from the yard made us jump. *My God! It's Robby's whistle!* By the time we reached the door, the whistle was blowing at a feverish pace. Visions of a rattlesnake filled my head as we raced into the yard. When we reached him, Robby was pointing frantically skyward, and we couldn't pry the whistle from his grip.

Looking up, we saw the most magnificent sight. Rain clouds—gigantic rain clouds with black, ominous bottoms!

"Robby! Help me, quickly! We need all the pots and pans from the kitchen!"

The whistle dropped from his lips and he raced with me to the house. Tom ran for the barn to drag out an old washtub. When all the containers were placed in the yard, Robby ran back to the house. He emerged with three wooden spoons from my kitchen drawer and handed one to each of us. He picked up my big stock pot and sat down cross-legged. Turning it over, he began to beat a rhythm with his spoon. Tom and I each reached for a pot and joined in.

"Rain for Robby! Rain for Robby!" I chanted with each beat.

A drop of water splashed on my pot and then another. Soon the yard was enveloped in soaking, glorious rain. We all stood with faces held upward to feel the absolute luxury of it. Tom picked up Robby and danced about the pots, shouting and whooping. That's when I heard it—softly at first—then louder and louder: the most marvelous, boisterous, giggling laughter. Tom swung about to show me Robby's face. With head tilted back, he was laughing right out loud! I hugged them both, tears of joy mixing with the rain. Robby released his grip from Tom and clutched my neck.

"W-W-Wobby's!" he stammered. Stretching out one tiny cupped hand to catch the downpour, he giggled again. "Wobby's . . . wain . . . Mom," he whispered.

Toni Fulco

A Dance with Dad

I am dancing with my father at my parents' fiftieth wedding anniversary. The band is playing an old-fashioned waltz as we move gracefully across the floor. His hand on my waist is as guiding as it always was, and he hums the tune to himself in a steady, youthful way. Around and around we go, laughing and nodding to the other dancers. We are the best dancers on the floor, they tell us. My father squeezes my hand and smiles at me.

As we continue to dip and sway, I remember a time when I was almost three and my father came home from work, swooped me into his arms and began to dance me around the table. My mother laughed at us, told us dinner would get cold. But my father said, "She's just caught the rhythm of the dance! Dinner can wait!" And then he sang out, "Roll out the barrel, we'll have a barrel of fun," and I sang back, "Let's get those blues on the run." That night, he taught me to polka, waltz and foxtrot while dinner waited.

We danced through the years. When I was five, my father taught me to "shuffle off to Buffalo." Later we won a dance contest at a Campfire Girls Round-Up. Then we learned to jitterbug at the USO place downtown. Once my father caught on to the steps, he danced with everyone in the hall—the women passing out doughnuts, even the GI's. We all laughed and clapped our hands for my father, the dancer.

One night when I was fifteen, lost in some painful, adolescent mood, my father put on a stack of records and teased me to dance with him. "C'mon," he said, "let's get those blues on the run." I turned away from him and hugged my pain closer than before. My father put his hand on my shoulder and I jumped out of the chair, screaming, "Don't touch me! Don't touch me! I am sick and tired of dancing with you!" The hurt on his face did not escape me, but the words were out, and I could not call them back. I ran to my room sobbing hysterically.

We did not dance together after that night. I found other partners, and my father waited up for me after dances, sitting in his favorite chair, clad in his flannel pajamas. Sometimes he would be asleep when I came in, and I would wake him, saying, "If you were so tired, you should have gone to bed."

"No, no," he'd say. "I was just waiting for you."

Then we'd lock up the house and go to bed.

My father waited up for me all through my high school and college years, while I danced my way out of his life.

One night, shortly after my first child was born, my mother called to tell me my father was ill. "A heart problem," she said. "Now, don't come. It's three hundred miles. Besides, it would upset your father. We'll just have to wait. I'll let you know."

My father's tests showed some stress, but a proper diet restored him to good health. Little things, then, for a while. A disc problem in the back, more heart trouble, a lens implant for cataracts. But the dancing did not stop. My mother wrote that they had joined a dance club. "You remember how your father loves to dance."

Yes, I remembered. My eyes filled up with remembering.

When my father retired, we mended our way back together again; hugs and kisses were common when we visited each other. But my father did not ask me to dance. He danced with the grandchildren; my daughters knew how to waltz before they could read.

"One, two, three and one, two, three," my father would count out, "won't you come and waltz with me?" Sometimes my heart ached to have him say those words to me. But I knew my father was waiting for an apology from me, and I could never find the right words.

As the time for my parents' fiftieth anniversary approached, my brothers and I met to plan the party. My older brother said, "Do you remember that night you wouldn't dance with him? Boy, was he mad! I couldn't believe he'd get so mad about a thing like that. I'll bet you haven't danced with him since."

I did not tell him he was right.

My younger brother promised to get the band.

"Make sure they can play waltzes and polkas," I told him.

"Dad can dance to anything," he said. "Don't you want to get down, get funky?" I did not tell him that all I wanted to do was dance once more with my father.

When the band began to play after dinner, my parents took the floor. They glided around the room, inviting the others to join them. The guests rose to their feet, applauding the golden couple. My father danced with his granddaughters, and then the band began to play the "Beer Barrel Polka."

"Roll out the barrel," I heard my father sing. Then I knew it was time. I knew the words I must say to my father before he would dance with me once more. I wound my way through a few couples and tapped my daughter on the shoulder.

"Excuse me," I said, almost choking on my words, "but I believe this is my dance."

My father stood rooted to the spot. Our eyes met and traveled back to that night when I was fifteen. In a trembling voice, I sang, "Let's get those blues on the run."

My father bowed and said, "Oh, yes. I've been waiting for you."

Then he started to laugh, and we moved into each other's arms, pausing for a moment so we could catch once more the rhythm of the dance.

Jean Jeffrey Gietzen

A Miracle of Love

My grandson, Daniel, and I have always been very close. When Daniel's father remarried after a divorce, Daniel, who was eleven, and his little sister, Kristie, came to live with us. My husband and I were more than happy to have kids in the house again.

Things were going along just fine until the diabetes I've lived with most of my adult life started affecting my eyes, and then more seriously, my kidneys. Then everything seemed to fall apart.

Three times a week, I had to go to the hospital to be hooked up to a dialysis machine. I was living, but I couldn't really call it a life—it was an existence. I had no energy. I dragged myself through my daily chores and slept as much as I could. My sense of humor seemed to disappear.

Daniel, seventeen by then, was really affected by the change in me. He tried as hard as he could to make me laugh, to bring back the grandma who loved to clown around with him. Even in my sorry state, Daniel could still bring a smile to my face.

But things were not improving. After a year on dialysis,

my condition was deteriorating and the doctors felt that if I didn't receive a kidney transplant within six months, I would surely die. No one told Daniel this, but he knew—he said all he had to do was look at me. To top it off, as my condition worsened, there was a chance I would become too weak to have the transplant surgery at all, and then there would be nothing they could do for me. So we started the tense and desperate wait for a kidney.

I was adamant that I didn't want a kidney from anyone I knew. I would wait until an appropriate kidney became available, or I would literally die waiting. But Daniel had other plans. The times that he took me to my dialysis appointments, he did a little secret research on his own. Then he announced his intentions to me.

"Grandma, I'm giving you one of my kidneys. I'm young and I'm healthy. . . . He paused. He could see I wasn't at all happy with his offer. He continued, almost in a whisper, "And most of all, I couldn't stand it if you weren't around." His face wore an expression of appeal mixed with determination. He can be as stubborn as a mule once he decides on something—but I've been told many times that I can out-stubborn any mule!

We argued. I couldn't let him do it. We both knew that if he gave up his kidney, he'd also give up his life's dream: to play football. That boy ate, drank and slept football. It was all he ever talked about. And he was good, too. Daniel was co-captain and star defensive tackle of his high school team; he expected to apply for a football scholarship and was looking forward to playing college football. He just loved the sport.

"How can I let you throw away the thing that means the most to you?" I pleaded with him.

"Grandma," he said softly, "compared to your life, football means nothing to me."

After that, I couldn't argue anymore. So we agreed to

see if he was a good donor match, and then we'd discuss it further. When the tests came back, they showed Daniel was a perfect match. That was it. I knew I wasn't going to win that argument, so we scheduled the transplant.

Both surgeries went smoothly. As soon as I came out of the anesthesia, I could tell things were different. I felt great! The nurses in the intensive care unit had to keep telling me to lie back and be quiet—I wasn't supposed to be that lively! I was afraid to go to sleep, for fear I would break the spell and wake up the way I had been before. But the good feeling didn't go away, and I spent the evening joking and laughing with anyone who would listen. It was so wonderful to feel alive again!

The next day, they moved me out of ICU and onto the floor where Daniel was recuperating three doors away. His grandfather helped him walk down to see me as soon as I was moved into my room. When we saw each other, we didn't know what to say. Holding hands, we just sat there and looked at each other for a long time, over-whelmed by the deep feeling of love that connected us.

Finally, he spoke. "Was it worthwhile, Grandma?"

I laughed a little ruefully. "It was for me! But was it for you?" I asked him.

He nodded and smiled at me. "I've got my grandma back."

And I have my life back. It still amazes me. Every morning, when I wake up, I thank God—and Daniel—for this miracle. A miracle born of the purest love.

Shirlee Allison

[EDITORS' NOTE: *As a result of Daniel's selfless gift, he was chosen as the nation's Most Coura-geous Student Athlete and flown to Disney World for the awards ceremony. While there, he met Bobby Bowden, coach of Florida State University's football team, the Seminoles. Daniel told Coach Bowden that he was an avid Seminoles fan and that it had always been his dream to be a Seminole. Bowden was so moved by this that he decided to make the young man's dream come true. At the time of this writing, Daniel is a student at FSU—on a full scholarship—and is a trainer for the univer-sity's football team, a highly valued member of the Seminoles.*]

A Dream Come True

They called it "A Dream Come True." The staff at Air Canada had been soliciting funds and donations for a year to take a planeful of kids to Disney World for a day, and this was the day. It was earlier, of course, than any day has a right to begin—4:00 A.M.

I scraped the frost from my windshield and started the car. The Children's Aid Society, where I worked, had been offered places for ten children in the Dream Come True flight, and we'd selected ten children, most of them in foster care, with backgrounds of poverty, neglect and abuse—children who would never otherwise get to see the Magic Kingdom. In my bag, I had the legal documents for each child, documents that with their formal language hid the reality of the traumas these young children had experienced.

We hoped that this trip would give them a glimpse into a brighter world, give them a chance to have one day of feeling special and having fun.

The chaos as we gathered at the airport before dawn was incredible. Each child was given a backpack stuffed with donated gifts, and the level of excitement was indescribable. A little girl with two brown braids asked me shyly if she could really keep the T-shirt in her backpack.

"This is all yours to keep," I explained, showing her the contents of her backpack.

"Forever?" she asked me.

"Forever," I said, and she rewarded me with a beaming smile. Several of the children rushed to the washrooms and put on their new clothes over the clothes they were already wearing. I couldn't convince them that they'd be too hot with all those layers once we reached Florida. Two little girls found a travel checker game among their gifts and plopped themselves down in the middle of the airport floor to play.

Then there was Corby. He was one of the older children, almost twelve, and he looked cynically at the other children who were almost bouncing around the room. Corby sat on a chair, his arms folded, his backpack tossed on the floor.

When I walked over to him, he just looked at me without saying a word.

"What's the matter, Corby?" I asked. I'd seen his file. I knew he'd been abused and repeatedly abandoned by a mother who breezed in and out of his life as it suited her. I don't think anyone was sure who his father was, least of all Corby. But it's painful to see someone so young look so cynical.

"Nothing." He looked around. "What's really happening, anyway?"

"You know what's happening. First, we're having breakfast. Then we get on the airplane and spend the day at Disney World."

"Right." He shook his head and turned away.

"Corby, it's the truth."

He didn't believe me. Before I could say anything else, the Air Canada staff began handing out juice and muffins, and I found myself busily mopping up spills and making sure everyone got enough to eat. Soon after, we followed the path of stars that had been put in place to guide us to the right plane, and I almost forgot my conversation with Corby as I settled the kids into their seats.

As I sat down, though, I found Corby right beside me.

"So," he said, "we're really going on an airplane."

"I told you."

"Where are you really taking us?"

"Corby, we are really, truly going to Disney World."

He shook his head again, clearly beginning to think that I was as foolish as the excited children around him. I, too, had been duped.

None of the kids in our group had ever been on an airplane before, so the trip was almost as exciting as Disney World itself. Everyone had a turn to sit by the window, to visit the pilot in the cockpit, and to order drinks or treats. Before long, we were on the ground again and emerging into ninety-degree Florida weather.

I could tell Corby was stunned. He grabbed one of the airport staff helping to unload the plane. "Is this really Florida?" he asked. The man in coveralls laughed and assured him that this was, indeed, Florida.

As we loaded the children onto the bus that took us to Disney World, Corby hung back. He wanted to sit with me again.

After a long silence, he said to me, "I know what's going to happen. You're going to leave us here, aren't you?"

"No, we're not. We're going to Disney World now, and then tonight, we're going home."

"And do I get to go back to the Mullins?" The Mullins were his foster parents, who had shown this often very difficult boy a great deal of love.

"Yes, you'll go back to the Mullins. I bet they'll be waiting at the airport when we land."

"Right." He didn't believe me about this, either.

The Magic Kingdom worked its magic. All the kids got Mickey Mouse ears, rode every ride once and many of them twice, stuffed themselves with quite unhealthy food, talked to Snow White and Minnie Mouse and all the other characters, clapped loudly at all the shows, and in general had a perfect day. It was exhausting for the adults, trying to keep track of our overexcited charges, but we didn't lose a single child. Not even Corby, who began to smile a little the second time he went through "It's a Small World" and who loved the Haunted Mansion almost as much as I did.

As darkness began to fall over the Magic Kingdom, we rounded up the children in our groups and gave each child a twenty-dollar bill. This was for buying souvenirs in the Main Street gift shops, so that each child could have a personal reminder of this special day.

But this was where I saw a new kind of magic. First the little girl with braids said to me, "I want to buy something for my brother because he didn't get to come. What do you think he'd like?" I helped her find a Mickey Mouse hat and yo-yo. Then another child asked for help in picking a gift for "this girl in my foster home who really wanted to come but she couldn't." And another wanted to purchase a gift for the teacher who had given him extra help all year.

So it went, one child after another. My eyes blurred with tears as each of these children—children who had been chosen for this trip because they came from impoverished, traumatic backgrounds—searched for the right gift for someone who had been left behind. Given a little money to spend as they chose, they spent it on others.

Finally, there was Corby.

"Are we really going home?" he asked me once more, but this time he was smiling and confident that he knew the answer.

"We're really, really going home," I told him.

"In that case," he said, "I'm going to buy presents for the Mullins."

I told him I thought that was a lovely idea and walked away before he saw me cry.

Teresa Pitman

Safe-Keeping

"I'm so glad you're coming to live with us, Aunt Emma," twelve-year-old Jane said as she placed a hand-knitted bunting into Emma's trunk of keepsakes. Jane and her mother were helping Aunt Emma pack in preparation for her move. Mama had gone downstairs to box up Aunt Emma's kitchen, leaving Jane upstairs to help Emma pack her sentimental items.

Jane stopped what she was doing for a minute and gazed out the open window of Emma's two-story farmhouse. She saw the roof of her own home, which stood at the far end of the cornfield. The wind carried the pounding of her father's hammer as he proudly finished the construction of additions to their new home, complete with extra rooms for Emma.

Emma sighed. "This old house is too big for me to ramble around in now that I'm all alone."

Young Jane's face reflected the anguish she saw on Emma's. It was still hard to believe Emma's husband and four children wouldn't come racing up the steps again. There were gone forever, all dying in one week during the last year's diphtheria epidemic.

Jane missed Emma's children more than anyone guessed. They had been like brothers and sisters to her. As an only child, she had spent most of her life ganging up with the two girls to fend off their two older, pesky brothers. Now, she usually cried as she walked home through the corn rows that had once been paths linking their lives.

"I'm really going to miss this old place, though." Emma waved her hand toward the faded wallpaper and worn woodwork. "This is the only home I've known since we left the old country."

Her eyes filled with tears as she hugged a baby quilt to her chest before placing it in the trunk.

"Tell me again about leaving Ireland with Mama and Papa," Jane coaxed, hoping to see Emma's eyes dance as usual when she recalled that adventure.

"You've heard that story a hundred times," Emma said, as she eased into the rocking chair with a bundle of children's clothes in her lap.

"But I love it!" Jane begged. "Tell me again about Mama and Papa then."

While she never gave much thought to having been adopted, Jane sometimes wondered whether that explained her relentless yearning for old family stories. She sat on the braided rug at the foot of the rocker and listened.

"Well, your mother and I were best friends—like sisters—all our lives."

Jane blurted in on cue, "That's why I call you Aunt, even though we're not related!"

Emma winked and smiled.

The truth was, next to Mama and Papa, Jane loved Emma more than anyone else in the world.

"So, of course, then our husbands became best friends," Emma continued.

"We did everything together, the four of us. We danced . . ." Emma's voice trailed off and her head swayed slightly, as if in time with the music. Then her eyes danced, too.

"We shared everything, good times and bad. Your mama was there at every one of our children's births, even though she could never give birth to a child of her own." Emma took her usual pause and shook her head slowly.

"There was never a woman who wanted or deserved a child more than your mama did. She wanted a baby more than anything else on earth."

"I know," Jane whispered, then beamed. "That's why I'm so glad she got me! She calls me her special gift."

Emma took a deep breath. "So when my husband, Patrick, had a chance to come to a Wisconsin farm in America, it didn't take long to decide your folks would come along, too. Like I said, we shared everything."

Emma rocked as she recounted the difficult journey. The storm at sea had tossed the ship for weeks longer than expected. All the passengers got sick.

"Especially me," Emma moaned. "I was expecting our fifth child. If it hadn't been for your mama, I wouldn't have survived that trip. Patrick and the others were far too sick to care for me. I could tell I was about to lose the baby." She stopped to blot tears with the child's shirt she was holding. "Your mother left her own sick bed to help me . . ." Her voice trailed off again. "She was an angel. If it hadn't been for her, both the baby and I would have died, then and there."

Jane rested her head on Emma's lap. "I'm so glad you made it. My life wouldn't have been the same without you."

Jane looked up into Emma's face. She knew that this was the part of the story that was hard for Emma to repeat, so Jane said it for her. "Thanks to Mama, that baby girl was born on that old ship, all pink and pretty!" Both their faces lit up—then faded when Jane added, "But the next day your baby went to live with the angels."

Emma only nodded, then abruptly stood and began placing the items on her lap into the trunk of treasures. Without speaking, she went to a bureau drawer and began sorting more children's clothes. Some worn items were put in a wooden crate. Others she placed reverently into the trunk.

The old wooden stairs creaked as Mama came up from the kitchen, took Jane's hand, and sat next to her on the bed.

From the bottom drawer, Emma retrieved a bundle wrapped in white linen and tied with a satin bow. She took it to the bed and unwrapped it slowly. One by one, she laid the tiny white garments on the bedspread.

"These are the baptism gowns I made for each of my babies before they were born," she said softly.

Mama squeezed Jane's hand.

Emma's fingers trembled as she smoothed the fabric and straightened the lace on each delicate gown. "I stitched each one by hand and crocheted the trim myself."

Mama reached for Emma's hand and stroked it, as if they both knew now was the time to tell me the *whole* story.

Emma picked up the gowns one at a time. "I was to give them to my children to keep when they grew up." She could barely speak. "This one was Colin's. This one was Shane's. This was Kathleen's. This was Margaret's."

Her tears fell onto the fifth one as she handed it to Jane. "And this one was yours."

Thoughts, memories and old stories tumbled wildly in Jane's head. She stared into her mama's eyes before turning back to Emma.

"What are you saying, Aunt Emma?"

Emma's voice shook. "Did you ever notice I never said that baby girl died, just that she went to live with God's angels?"

Jane nodded. "I was that baby?" Her lips curved in a hesitant smile. "And Mama and Papa were God's angels on earth!"

Now Emma nodded. "It was tradition in the old country, when someone couldn't have a baby, another family would give them one of theirs. I loved your mama so much. . . . Her voice broke, so Mama finished the sentence. "She and Patrick gave us the greatest gift of love."

Jane's smile widened. "Your special gift." She wrapped her arms around her mama.

Tears flooded down Mama's cheeks as she rocked Jane in her arms. "It's as if God gave you to Papa and me for safe-keeping."

Emma cried softly, "Oh Jane . . . I'd have lost you with the others."

Jane fondled the baptism gown in her hands, then embraced Emma, whispering, "Thank you."

The sound of Papa's hammering drifted through the open window. Emma smiled and her eyes danced. "Twelve years ago on that ship, I gave your folks the greatest gift. Now they share that special gift with me."

LeAnn Thieman

The Best Badge of All

When I became a Girl Scout, my mother told me this story about her scout troop and what happened to them a long time ago, during World War II:

> On a chilly Saturday morning in December, the eleven-year-old girls in our troop gathered excitedly at the bus stop, where we met our leader, Mrs. Taylor. We carried large paper sacks filled with skillets, mixing bowls and assorted groceries. On this long-awaited day, the girls of Troop 11 were going to earn our cooking badges.
>
> "Nothing tastes as good as the first meal you cook yourself, especially on an open fire," Mrs. Taylor smiled.
>
> It would take three bus transfers to get us all the way out to the wilderness. As we boarded the first, we clutched our groceries as if they were bags of jewels. Several mothers had generously contributed precious ration stamps so we could buy the ingredients for a real breakfast: pancakes with actual butter, bacon, and even some brown sugar for homemade syrup! We scouts would earn our badges in spite of hardship, in spite of

the war. In our minds, we were not only learning to cook in the wilderness; we were doing our parts to keep life going apace on the home front.

We finally arrived at Papango Park, a beautiful desert refuge filled with palo verde trees, smoky mesquite bushes and massive red rock formations. As we started hiking up the dirt road into the park, a U.S. Army truck filled with German prisoners of war passed us, heading into the park.

"There go those Germans!" one of the girls said, contemptuously. "I hate them!"

"Why did they have to start the war?" another complained. "My dad's been gone for so long."

We all had fathers, brothers or uncles fighting in Europe.

Determinedly, we hiked to our campsite, and soon the bacon was sizzling in the skillets while the pancakes turned golden brown around the edges.

The meal was a success. Mrs. Taylor's prediction about our gastronomic delight was proved correct.

After the meal, one of the girls started a scouting song as we cleaned up our cooking site. One by one, we all joined in. Our leader started another song, and we continued wholeheartedly.

Then, unexpectedly, we heard male voices. A beautiful tune sung in deep, strong tones filled the December air and drifted down to us.

We looked up to see the cavernous natural shell in the red sediment boulders, called "Hole in the Rock," filled with the German prisoners and their guards.

As they finished their song, we began another. They reciprocated with another haunting melody. We couldn't understand a word they were singing, but to our delight, we continued exchanging songs throughout the clear desert morning.

Finally one of the girls began to sing "Silent Night," and we all added our voices to the Christmas carol. A few moments of silence followed, and then ... the familiar melody flowed back to us.

"Stille Nacht, Heilige Nacht ... "

"How can they know our Christmas carols?" one of the girls asked our leader. They were our country's enemies!

We continued to listen in awe. For an odd, unforgettable moment, the men in the cave became somebody's fathers and brothers, just as they understood us to be beloved daughters and sisters.

In the years that followed, others probably looked at our new badges as proof that we could cook over a fire. But to us, they were reminders of the need for peace, and a very strange transformation that happened one Christmastime.

Gerry Niskern

The Christmas Star

This was my grandmother's first Christmas without Grandfather, and we had promised him before he passed away that we would make this her best Christmas ever. When my mom, dad, three sisters and I arrived at her little house in the Blue Ridge Mountains of North Carolina, we found she had waited up all night for us to arrive from Texas. After we exchanged hugs, Donna, Karen, Kristi and I ran into the house. It did seem a little empty without Grandfather, and we knew it was up to us to make this Christmas special for her.

Grandfather had always said that the Christmas tree was the most important decoration of all. So we immediately set to work assembling the beautiful artificial tree that was stored in Grandfather's closet. Although artificial, it was the most genuine-looking Douglas fir I had ever seen. Tucked away in the closet with the tree was a spectacular array of ornaments, many of which had been my father's when he was a little boy. As we unwrapped each one, Grandmother had a story to go along with it. My mother strung the tree with bright white lights and a red button garland; my sisters and I carefully placed the ornaments on the tree; and finally, Father was given the honor of lighting the tree.

We stepped back to admire our handiwork. To us, it looked magnificent, as beautiful as the tree in Rockefeller Center. But something was missing.

"Where's your star?" I asked.

The star was my grandmother's favorite part of the tree.

"Why, it must be here somewhere," she said, starting to sort through the boxes again. "Your grandfather always packed everything so carefully when he took the tree down."

As we emptied box after box and found no star, my grandmother's eyes filled with tears. This was no ordinary ornament, but an elaborate golden star covered with colored jewels and blue lights that blinked on and off. Moreover, Grandfather had given it to Grandmother some fifty years ago, on their first Christmas together. Now, on her first Christmas without him, the star was gone, too.

"Don't worry, Grandmother," I reassured her. "We'll find it for you."

My sisters and I formed a search party.

"Let's start in the closet where the ornaments were," Donna said. "Maybe the box just fell down."

That sounded logical, so we climbed on a chair and began to search that tall closet of Grandfather's. We found Father's old yearbooks and photographs of relatives, Christmas cards from years gone by, and party dresses and jewelry boxes, but no star.

We searched under beds and over shelves, inside and outside, until we had exhausted every possibility. We could see Grandmother was disappointed, although she tried not to show it.

"We could buy a new star," Kristi offered.

"I'll make you one from construction paper," Karen chimed in.

"No," Grandmother said. "This year, we won't have a star."

By now, it was dark outside, and time for bed, as Santa would soon be here. We lay in bed, snowflakes falling quietly outside.

The next morning, my sisters and I woke up early, as was our habit on Christmas day—first, to see what Santa had left under the tree, and second, to look for the Christmas star in the sky. After a traditional breakfast of apple pancakes, the family sat down together to open presents. Santa had brought me the Easy-Bake Oven I wanted, and Donna a Chatty-Cathy doll. Karen was thrilled to get the doll buggy she had asked for, and Kristi to get the china tea set. Father was in charge of passing out the presents, so that everyone would have something to open at the same time.

"The last gift is to Grandmother from Grandfather," he said, in a puzzled voice.

"From who?" There was surprise in my grandmother's voice.

"I found that gift in Grandfather's closet when we got the tree down," Mother explained. "It was already wrapped so I put it under the tree. I thought it was one of yours."

"Hurry and open it," Karen urged excitedly.

My grandmother shakily opened the box. Her face lit up with joy when she unfolded the tissue paper and pulled out a glorious golden star. There was a note attached. Her voice trembled as she read it aloud:

> *Don't be angry with me, dear. I broke your star while putting away the decorations, and I couldn't bear to tell you. Thought it was time for a new one. I hope it brings you as much joy as the first one. Merry Christmas.*
>
> *Love,*
> *Bryant*

So Grandmother's tree had a star after all, a star that expressed my grandparents' everlasting love for one another. It brought my grandfather home for Christmas in each of our hearts and made it our best Christmas ever.

Susan Adair

My Dad, Charlie and Me

My father's long and successful career began in the days of vaudeville. The famous ventriloquist, Edgar Bergen and his equally famous wooden sidekick, Charlie McCarthy, delighted theater and later, radio and television audiences for decades. So when I was born, it was only natural that I was known in the press not as Candice Bergen, but as "Charlie's sister." As a little girl, I sometimes performed with Daddy and Charlie. I recited my well-learned lines with considerable poise and polish—a daughter determined to make good.

Many years later, in the summer of 1978, my father called a press conference at the Brown Derby in Beverly Hills to announce his retirement, half-wondering whether anyone would show up. He was surprised when the press conference, packed, was carried on the evening news.

His final appearance, he announced, would be a three-week engagement at Caesar's Palace in Las Vegas on a bill with Andy Williams. This was a serious risk for a man who, not six months before, had been hospitalized in coronary intensive care. But as soon as the offer had been made, he was hellbent on accepting it, determined, one last time, to "play the Palace on the top of the bill": Edgar Bergen and Charlie McCarthy just like way back when. Here was an opportunity to go out in style.

My mother went with him to Las Vegas, and on opening night my brother Kris and I were there to surprise him. We were sitting out front as the lights dimmed and the music started up, hoping he would make it smoothly through the routines, terrified that he might not.

The three of us barely breathed as the orchestra led into "Charlie My Boy," the familiar theme brought into America's living rooms by radio thirty years before. There were many there that night who remembered—people for whom Edgar and Charlie were old fireside friends—and as Bergen walked from the wings with McCarthy at his side, the applause was long and alive with memories.

My father stood straight and proud on the stage, his right hand on Charlie's back. For this occasion, his final farewell, he had insisted on playing again in white tie and tails. He was, after all, an elegant man, a poised and graceful presence commanding center stage.

"Well, Charlie—"

"Bergen, you old windbag, I'll kill ya, so help me, I'll mooowwww you down—"

And they slipped into the familiar patter of a partnership that had lasted sixty years.

The routine was flawless. Bergen reasoning, McCarthy saucy and razzing, the steady laughter of the audience, the frequent applause. Nothing could stop them, and the audience kept asking for more.

My mother sat still as a statue, her concentration locked on the man on the stage. Only her lips moved as she unconsciously mouthed the dialogue she had followed for thirty-five years, as if willing it to come out right. Each of us knew by heart the lines of the routines that had spanned our lives; but that night we heard them fresh, as if for the first time—

perhaps because we sensed it would be the last.

The act ended with a sound track from their old radio shows, a montage of Bergen and McCarthy memories: John Barrymore jousting with Charlie; Marilyn Monroe and Charles McCarthy announcing their engagement; W. C. Fields threatening to split Charlie into Venetian blinds—flashbacks of famous voices from the past. Up on stage, Edgar and Charlie cocked their heads, swapped knowing glances and chuckled softly as they looked up, listening wistfully to their lives.

Then my father said simply, "In vaudeville, every act has to have a close, and I think, for me, the close has come and it's time to pack up my little friend and say good-bye. Goodnight, God bless, and thank you all for listening." As the orchestra played his favorite, "September Song," he picked up Charlie and walked offstage.

The three of us smiled and cried, trying to compose ourselves before the house lights came up. The audience rose to its feet, applauding him with deep affection, grateful to share his farewell.

There were photographers in his dressing room backstage as we entered, and we had to press our way through the throng. He hugged Kris and my mother; then I came forward, wiping my eyes. We held each other tight. The love of a lifetime was squeezed into those moments. Once again I started sobbing, so proud of him, so happy for him, so sad. Knowing somehow that it was a last good-bye. His to an audience, ours to him.

The reviews of the show were unanimous, effusive in their praise. The next three days' performances went just as smoothly, with standing ovations at the end of each.

After the fourth night's performance, my father went to sleep in good spirits. My mother rose early, half opened the blinds and called to him. Several moments passed before she realized he was dead. He had gone peacefully while he slept.

For my father, there could have been no better ending; it was one he might have written himself. And who can say that he hadn't? There was the supreme sense of timing ingrained over sixty years of performing. Just as in vaudeville, he knew when to close.

Candice Bergen

My Dad

Whenever anyone meets my dad, I imagine they first notice how handsome he is: the striking blue eyes, jet black hair and cleft in his chin. But next, I'll bet they notice his hands. He's a professional carpenter; he usually has a bruised nail or two, several fresh cuts, various healing wounds and calluses everywhere. The girth of his fingers is three times the size of an average man's finger. They are the hands of a man who started his working life at the early age of three, milking cows. His attitude toward a work crew can appear gruff; he expects them to work hard and do whatever it takes to finish the job without excuses.

Twenty-three years ago, my mom died, and this man's man was left all alone to raise a fourteen-year-old girl and an eleven-year-old boy. He suddenly had to be Dad *and* Mom.

It seemed easier at first. I was a rather fearless child and preferred playing with boys, doing boy things like climbing trees, building forts, playing football, baseball and with G.I. Joes. I did have a Barbie doll, but she often wore G.I. Joe fatigues and went to war with him. I even played on an all-boys' ice hockey team. I had a lot of fun and learned many things from these activities. But none of them prepared me for stepping into my womanhood, which had to happen sooner or later.

I especially remember one day when I was about fifteen years old. We were driving down to Georgia to visit my aunt, and for some reason, every single thing my dad and my brother said or did made me crazy! I went from weepy to laughing for no reason, but my overall desire was to be *left alone!* It was clear they were both perplexed by this Jekyll/Hyde creature in their car.

We'd been taking our time driving and ended up spending the night at a motor lodge along the highway. Once we were in the room, Dad sent my brother out to the soda machine. When we were alone, he asked me what was wrong. There was nothing to do but admit that I'd begun menstruating for the very first time in my life. Then I burst out crying uncontrollably.

The miracle was that somehow, even though no booklet included this piece of information, Dad knew to just hold me and allow me to mourn the loss of my childhood.

He then offered to go to the store for me and buy the items I required.

We both crossed some kind of bridge that day: me into womanhood and he more deeply into the role of being mother as well as father. I think some men fear their feminine side, as if being nurturing would take away from their manliness somehow. All my dad knew to do was to love me unconditionally; not surprisingly, that worked just fine.

When my senior prom rolled around, I found myself in the happy position of dating a boy from a neighboring town; we invited each other to our proms, which were on consecutive nights.

Daddy wanted to make certain I had the perfect dress, and I did. It was a sleeveless, long white eyelet gown with a scoop neck. It made me feel like a princess. And Dad's approval was obvious; I think he was proud of me for stepping out of my tomboy image and acting the young lady—even if only for a couple of nights.

But what nights they were! Tradition at our school's prom was to stay out all night with your friends. With our parents' permission, my date and I "prommed" until 6:30 in the morning. I returned to my home to sleep for a few hours before driving to his parents' house.

I'll never forget my amazement that Saturday morning when I awoke and came downstairs to find my beautiful prom gown proudly displayed in protective plastic, like new, ready for another night's festivities.

It seems that sometime during my sleep, my dad had come into my room and found my prom gown. He had hand-washed it in a delicate laundry soap, then hand-pressed it.

My dad may not have been a man of many words when he was raising us, but he didn't really have to be. When I think of those beat-up working man's callused hands gently washing my delicate prom gown, my heart warms and relives that moment of unconditional love all over again.

It felt like the best of what we're supposed to learn from our mothers—and our dads.

Barbara E. C. Goodrich

A Happy-Ever-After

"Is this Jenna?" the voice on the phone asked.

Jenna clutched the receiver with a trembling hand. That voice was exactly as she had dreamed it would sound. Just exactly like his father's.

Jenna had known for thirty years that this day would come. Adopted children seem to want to know all about their natural families. Feelings of dread, but a sort of elation, filled Jenna while she carried on a conversation with the young man on the phone.

In 1967, Jenna was in love with David. But David's family was from the poorer section of town. Jenna's father was controlling and abusive, and he would not allow her to date David. With the help of friends, they sneaked around to see each other.

When Jenna discovered that she was pregnant, her father became enraged. He forced the teen to go away to live with an aunt until the baby was born. Heartbroken, David joined the army and went to fight in Vietnam. He wrote some letters to Jenna, but her father threw them away. David even tried writing letters to one of Jenna's friends, hoping to get some word to the girl he dearly loved. Jenna never received any of the letters, and she didn't know how to contact David.

Jenna came home after the baby was born. She dreamed constantly of the tiny infant she had held for only a second. She wondered what his adoptive parents were like, where they lived, and what the baby was growing to look like. She also dreamed of the day she would be old enough to leave home and get away from her controlling father. After graduation, Jenna went to college, then got a good job in a large city. She never returned to her hometown, still angry that her father had not allowed her to keep her child and marry David.

Memories of a lost love and a son she had to give away caused Jenna to never marry. She kept busy with her job as a school teacher. Organizations for battered women and unwed mothers became her passion. Jenna worked very hard to help others all her adult life.

But in the back of her mind, she always knew that this day would come. Her son would find her and want to know why she hadn't loved him enough to keep him.

"Can we meet sometime soon?" the young man asked. His name was Bradley. Jenna agreed to allow him to fly to her city and meet her. He was thirty years old and married. He had two children.

After she hung up, Jenna wished she had asked if Bradley had been able to find David. She let the thought die and began to prepare for the visit from her son in two weeks.

The days dragged. Jenna's emotions flew. She went from excitement at seeing her son at last, to dread that he wouldn't like her or wouldn't understand.

Finally, the day arrived. Jenna drove to the airport two hours early because she was too nervous to stay home alone. She paced and bit her nails.

Bradley's flight was announced. Jenna got as close to

the gate as she was allowed, craning her neck to watch for the family she was about to claim. A lifetime of nightmares and regrets filled her mind.

Suddenly, there he was, right in front of her. A hug so tight that he picked her up was the first touch from her son in thirty years. They hugged and cried for several minutes. Then a little boy tugged at Bradley's shirt.

"Daddy, I'm thirsty." Jenna hugged her grandson, then his older sister. She hugged her daughter-in-law, and then hugged Bradley some more. The little boy began to shout and run toward another man. "Grandpa!" he yelled.

Jenna stopped and stared. *It can't be. But how? Is it really him?*

Bradley dropped a soft kiss on Jenna's cheek. "Yes, it's really him. I found him last week, and he has been to the house to visit us. He was very excited to know that I was meeting you today. He's never married, either, you know."

David picked up the little boy, then his eyes met Jenna's. He gently put the boy down. In an instant, he reached Jenna. She was in his arms a long time before they pulled apart to look at each other.

The weekend ended much too soon. Bradley and his wife made Jenna promise to come visit in a few weeks. When they went to the airport, David helped Bradley's family get situated.

"Where are you flying out from?" Jenna asked.

"I'm not," he answered. "I've extended my vacation. We have a lot of years to make up for."

Bradley was able to witness his parents' marriage at Christmastime that year.

Yes, there really are some happily-ever-afters.

Mary J. Davis

Holding On

A friend may well be reckoned the masterpiece of nature.

Ralph Waldo Emerson

When I was a kid, I used to wake up, pull on jeans, and race down the street to Ann's house.

Today, I take my time getting ready. I walk around our old neighborhood, noticing the crepe myrtle bush Ann and I used to plunder, the magnolia trees still gracing the lawns, the sewer grate where Ann and I sat and practiced cussing.

I take a breath and knock on the door of Ann's house, where she's visiting her parents. Her father answers.

"She's in her room," he says.

The hallway seems smaller than I remembered.

"Come in," Ann says, to my timid knock. I look at the pictures lining the hall before I turn the knob—Ann with two missing front teeth, Ann wearing a frilly yellow dress and riding a pony, Ann wearing her graduation robe. In the years since we've seen each other, we've added careers, husbands, children to our lives. In the past five years, Ann has struggled with cancer.

Ann looks fragile and beautiful, posed among the bed's pillows. She wears a pink satin nightgown. A red scarf covers her head. A cigarette quivers in her right hand.

When she was fourteen, Ann would wake up and strike a match against the wall to light her first cigarette of the day. I loved seeing the charcoal streaks sweep her wall, like oriental symbols. Decadent, I thought enviously. Ann could do whatever she wanted and her father never got mad.

Ann's father comes into the room, bringing us cups of herbal tea.

"Do you need anything else?" he asks. Silver softens his once black hair.

Ann smiles and shakes her head. She pats the bed and I settle beside her, giving her a gentle hug. I hold her as if she is a secret unfolding.

"Guess what! I'm finally skinnier than you," she says, laughing and displaying legs that look childlike in their spindliness.

The morphine Ann takes so she can sit up without pain has softened her speech. Still, her giggle is the same. The round sweetness of her face is the same as when we were four years old and just becoming friends.

"Want to be best friends?" Ann had asked me. We stood across from each other, with a hedge between us. We had each just moved into the neighborhood.

"Sure," I said.

"Debbie, come in for dinner," my mother called for the second time.

I watched Ann walk down the street to her house, stooping to capture dandelions along the way. Then I skipped across the yard, the new grass nibbling my feet. I felt like a balloon at last released to the sky. Something important had happened: I was no longer dependent on my mother and father for love. I had a friend.

"Excuse me while I go to the bathroom," Ann says. She used to always beat me at relays. Now, she walks gingerly, as if she is holding eggs in her pocket.

I think of Ann and me as kids, cramming into the family bathroom, taking turns, one on the toilet, one perched on the side of the tub. Going to the bathroom was the same as playing jacks or dressing dolls. We saw no need to be separated.

Yet we have been separated for years, staying in touch when we need comfort and talk. Ann knows my daughters without having met them; I love her husband for the wondrous supportive way he nurtures her. I look around her old bedroom and see the bookshelf with old copies of *Little Women*, *The Royal Road to Romance*, *Catcher in the Rye*, *Atlas Shrugged*—books that wove a path through our girlhood.

"Would you like to see my head?" Ann asks, when she comes back into the room.

"Yes," I say.

I hold my breath as Ann pulls off her scarf. She looks luminescent without the covering. The powerful curve of her skull is softened by a few wildflower wisps of hair.

I touch my hair, remembering the hours of agony I spent rolling my hair on orange juice cans so I could have the same soft waves as Ann. Ann's dark hair always curled under in just the right way, while mine was a frenetic mass of frizz.

"At first, I was scared to walk around without the wig. But it turns out my husband likes me like this. I catch him looking at me and smiling," she says.

She slowly settles back in bed, and as we have done so many times, we talk. We used to talk about boys; now we discuss men. We used to talk about school; now we talk about work. We talked about who we wanted to be and the differences we yearned to make: We still do. Our history links us together, like charms on a silver bracelet.

Ann tells me about her year of terrifying pain, of not being able to eat, of wondering if she'd even be healthy enough to complete her chemotherapy. I am silenced by her courage, awed by her strength.

"Tell me about you," she insists. "Tell me about your daughters."

As I begin, I notice her eyes fluttering closed.

I too close my eyes. As girls we slept together in many different places: the backseat of our fathers' cars, her playhouse near the crabapple tree, my double bed, a blanket spread on the front lawn.

I wake up to feel a blanket being draped over me. Ann's dad is tucking me in. Ann is already covered with a soft maroon quilt.

"You were sleeping so peacefully," he whispers. "It reminded me of when you were girls."

I feel cozy and cared for. I watch my friend sleeping, her face a familiar song.

She opens her eyes and smiles at me.

"I wouldn't fall asleep in front of just anyone," she says.

"Me neither," I tell her.

I scoot closer and touch her wrist. I remember playing games of Red Rover, clasping hands and holding fast while kids tried to break through our grasp.

"Red Rover, Red Rover, can Billy come over," we chanted.

Billy bombarded our clasped hands, running fast, hurling himself hard at us. Somehow, we hung onto each other and did not let go.

Ann takes my hand. Pain tightens her face. I curl my fingers between hers and hold on tight.

Deborah Shouse

Of Miracles, Children and Joshua's Jingle Bell

Each year, around Christmas, I bring out a tiny symbol from the back corners of my desk. The red satin ribbon is faded and frayed, but the shiny bell still jingles. It always brings back memories of a very special child I knew when I was a kindergarten teacher in a Cleveland public school. It also reminds me of an important message I try to pass on to the new generation of educators: The powerful love of children can sometimes accomplish miracles.

I recall vividly how the winds from nearby Lake Erie could rattle the windowpanes in our kindergarten classroom. The school was a tall, imposing brick structure, in a neighborhood at the edge of an industrial area—not as barren or forbidding as the Flats, but still shabby and decayed. Pungent fumes from a paint factory wafted in on clear days. Banks of tall windows enclosed two sides of our room. The usual wooden cabinets held supplies.

My second year of teaching was memorable because my classroom overflowed with children—forty in the morning session and forty more in the afternoon. *How could I possibly manage one more,* I thought angrily, when the principal informed me, a few days after school began, that an additional youngster—a handicapped child—had been admitted.

Along with his registration form was a letter from a pediatrician, asking us to allow Joshua to participate in as many activities as his physical condition permitted, because more than anything he needed to be with children his own age. What could I say? Somehow I would have to manage.

The next morning, Joshua and his mother arrived. He was gnome-like. His head was enormous, and he had luminous black eyes, stretched out strangely at the corners. His mother gave him a last hug and kiss. The only tears were hers. Joshua's unusual face was lit up by a broad smile during most of the morning. Clearly, he was happy to be with other children. I wished I could match his happy mood.

Joshua's appearance was just one of his multiple handicaps. He had poor motor control, often stumbling over his own and other people's feet. Handling a paint brush was a tremendous task. He usually grasped it in a grubby fist and splattered away with great gusto. His art projects demanded strategy and diplomacy of us all. Someone always wanted to help him cut with the scissors or to finish his work for him. But he was very determined. He wanted to do it by himself.

His Thanksgiving turkey was a complete disaster. Multicolored tail feathers emerged where the head should have been. Globs of paste oozed out as he worked, dripping down onto the floor. Time for the Christmas program was drawing near, and I began to have uneasy feelings.

Cities like Cleveland, New York and Chicago are still home to a melange of ethnic groups. Our classroom that year was a modern-day example of the old melting pot. The majority of the children were Irish, making their solo excursion into public school before joining their brothers and sisters at the local parish school. We also had Greeks, Italians, Syrians, Lebanese, Germans, Hungarians and Chinese, as well as many migrants from Appalachia.

To my surprise, Joshua was accepted unconditionally by the children. The day we talked about where we were born, he was unusually animated. Why, he had been born at Lutheran Hospital, too, just like half the class. He was really one of them. He belonged.

We began to shape and polish our Christmas program. It was always a social event of the first magnitude. Parents took off from work. Mothers baked their special holiday cookies. There would be new dresses for the girls and trips to the barbershop for the boys.

There was one thing Joshua did do well. He could jingle his bell. The bells were threaded on thin red ribbons and decorated the children's wrists. We helped to tie each other's in a big bow, proud of the newly acquired skill. Someone was always nearby to help Joshua tie his. We shook our bells in unison, singing: "Jingle, jingle, jingle, Christmas bell. I've got a secret. Don't you tell! (Shh! Shh!) Santa's going to visit you and me. Let's all dance merrily."

Shuffle, slide, shuffle, slide. In a carefully rehearsed circle dance, there were many chances to jingle, jingle, jingle. Joshua's eyes sparkled. He loved to jingle his bell. The only problem was that he hated to stop. He would jingle-jingle away, long after everyone else had finished.

A glimmer of hope flickered in my mind—perhaps his mother would sense the difficult situation and keep him home. I hated myself for the cruel thought, but I rationalized that it would be for the good of the group.

I was very, very wrong.

The day before the program, I couldn't stand the suspense. I called his home and asked if he would be participating the next day. "Oh, yes!" his mother answered in her halting English. "He come!" The program would proceed . . . including Joshua.

The day was typical for Cleveland. Leaden gray skies heralded a cold, dismal day. It might be months before we saw the sun again. Inside our kindergarten room, though, warmth and love glowed over all. One young father came in overalls, straight from his factory job nearby. Bridget's dad came in his fireman's dress uniform, resplendent with polished brass buttons and shiny black shoes. Mary Chung's family had closed the laundry for the morning. The entire clan was there, including an ancient grandmother. Joshua's mother came with her married daughter.

As the frigid gusts howled outside, we warmed up with songs, singing of the Prince of Peace and of Santa on the rooftop. Joshua did quite well. At least, he did not fall down. There was always a helping hand stretched out at critical moments. His cheeks were flushed, his eyes shining. He was trying very hard. I found myself with an enormous lump in my throat. Tears blurred my eyes so that I could barely read the notes. Glancing over at Joshua's mother, I could see tears on her cheeks, too.

When it came time to perform our finale, "Jingle, Jingle, Jingle, Christmas Bell," Joshua was ready. He tinkled and shook his bell in all the right places. When forty other little fingers were placed on forty little lips in a much-rehearsed "Shh! Shh!" so were Joshua's. He was doing everything correctly, along with the other children. He was transformed for those brief moments, freed from the burden of his physical ills. The love and warmth of the children encased him like a cocoon, and a beautiful Joshua emerged. It was a Christmas miracle.

The cookies, sumptuous with honey, figs and sesame seeds, disappeared quickly. The parents were delighted with the program. The children were only five years old, yet they had given us the best gift of all—themselves.

I went back East to visit my mother for the holidays. When I returned to school in January, there was a letter in my mailbox. It was from Joshua's married sister, written for her mother. Joshua had died peacefully in his sleep, a few days after Christmas. The brief period he had spent in kindergarten had been the happiest in his life.

How could I possibly explain Joshua's death to the children? They had so little idea of life's final passage. Thinking they would understand a simple explanation best, I told them Joshua had gone to heaven.

"You mean," Michael piped up, "he went to be one of them Christmas angels?"

What a great idea, I thought. *God bless you, Michael.* Dozens of little heads nodded in agreement. Oh, yes! Our Joshua was a Christmas angel now!

Each year, when I hear the church bells ring out joyously at Christmas, I look at his little bell and think of Joshua. He taught all of us—especially me—what miracles the love of children can accomplish.

Aline Stomfay-Stitz
Submitted by Carol Repella

Love in Action

One night a man came to our house and told me, "There is a family with eight children. They have not eaten for days." I took some food with me and went.

When I finally came to that family, I saw the faces of those little children disfigured by hunger. There was no sorrow or sadness in their faces, just the deep pain of hunger.

I gave the rice to the mother. She divided the rice in two, and went out, carrying half the rice. When she came back, I asked her, "Where did you go?" She gave me this simple answer, "To my neighbors—they are hungry also!"

. . . I was not surprised that she gave, because poor people are really very generous. But I was surprised that she knew they were hungry. As a rule, when we are suffering, we are so focused on ourselves we have no time for others.

Mother Teresa

2

ON ATTITUDE

I will tell you that there have been no failures
in my life. I don't want to sound like some
metaphysical queen, but there have been no
failures. There have been some tremendous
lessons.

Oprah Winfrey

The True Spirit of Christmas

If you can't change your fate, change your attitude.

Amy Tan

One more hour, I thought. *Just one more hour and I'm free.* It was Christmas Eve and I was stuck in beauty college. It wasn't fair. I had better things to do than wait on fussy old women with blue hair. I had worked hard and fast to get four shampoo-sets and one manicure finished before lunch. If I had no more appointments scheduled, I could leave at two o'clock. Just one more . . .

"Number seventy-one. Carolyn, number seventy-one."

The receptionist's voice over the intercom made my heart fall to my stomach.

"You have a phone call."

A phone call. I exhaled a sigh of relief and headed up front to take the call.

As I reached for the phone, I gave the appointment pad a cursory glance to confirm my freedom. I couldn't believe it. I had a 4:30 perm. No one in her right mind would have her hair done on Christmas Eve. No one would be so inconsiderate.

I glared at the receptionist behind the counter. "How could you do this?"

She took a step backward and whispered, "Mrs. Weiman scheduled you." Mrs. Weiman was the senior instructor, the biddy of the ball. When she spoke, no one argued.

"Fine," I hissed and turned to the phone. It was Grant. His grandmother had invited me to Christmas Eve dinner, and could I be ready by three o'clock? I fingered the diamond snowflake necklace he had given me the night before. Swallowing the lump in my throat, I explained the situation. After an interminable silence, he said we'd make it another time and hung up. Tears stung my eyes as I slammed the phone down and barricaded myself behind my station.

The afternoon hung bleak and gray, echoing my mood. Most of the other students had gone home. I had no other patrons until the 4:30 perm, and I spent the time at my station, stewing.

At about 4:15, Mrs. Weiman stuck her pinched face around my mirror and advised me in her soft, no-nonsense tone, "Change your attitude before she gets here," then quietly stepped away.

My mood would change all right, from angry to murderous. I grabbed a tissue and whisked away the fresh tears.

My number was called at 4:45. My tardy, inconsiderate patron had arrived. I strode brusquely up front to greet a very shriveled, frail old woman gently supported by her husband. With a tender voice, Mrs. Weiman introduced me to Mrs. Sussman and began escorting her to my station. Mr. Sussman followed us, mumbling his apologies for bringing her in so late.

I was still feeling put upon, but I tried not to show it. Mrs. Weiman cradled Mrs. Sussman closely as she lowered her into my chair. When she began raising the hydraulic chair, I feigned a smile and took over, stepping on the foot pump. Mrs. Sussman was so small, I had to raise the chair to its full height.

I placed a towel and plastic drape around her shoulders, then jumped back, aghast. Lice and mites were crawling over her scalp and shoulders. As I stood there trying not to retch, Mrs. Weiman reappeared, pulling on plastic gloves.

Mrs. Sussman's gray top knot was so matted, we couldn't pull the hairpins out. It disgusted me to think anyone could be so unkempt. Mrs. Weiman explained that we'd have to cut her hair to get the mat out, and Mrs. Sussman just looked at us with tears streaming down her cheeks. Her husband held her hands tenderly in his as he knelt beside the chair.

"Her hair was her pride all of her life," he explained. "She put it up like that on the morning I took her to the nursing home."

Evidently her hair hadn't been combed or cleaned since that morning nearly a year before. His eyes misted over, and he shuffled to the waiting room.

Mrs. Weiman cut the matted top knot gently away, revealing a withered scalp peeling with yellow decay. She worked patiently and lovingly, and I feebly tried to help where I could. A perm would eat through her scalp like acid. It was out of the question. We bathed her scalp gently, trying to dislodge the lice without tearing her hair out. I dabbed antiseptic ointment on her festering sores and twisted her sparse hair into pincurls. The curls were held in place by gel, for we didn't dare scrape her scalp with clips. Then we gently fanned her curls dry near the warmth of the radiator.

Mrs. Sussman slipped a palsied hand into her tiny bag and drew out a tube of lipstick and a pair of white lace gloves. Mrs. Weiman dabbed the lipstick softly on her lips, then carefully threaded the shaking hands into the dainty gloves. My thoughts were drawn to my grandmother, who had recently passed away—how she always put on lipstick before walking to the mailbox on the curb. I thought of stories she told of her youth, when no proper lady would be seen in public without her gloves. Tears formed in my eyes as I silently thanked God for having taken her with dignity.

Mrs. Weiman left me to sterilize my station and returned with Mr. Sussman. When he saw his wife, their mutual tears flowed unchecked. "Oh, my dear," he whispered, "you've never looked lovelier."

Her lips trembled in a smile.

He reached into his coat pocket and presented Mrs. Weiman and me each with a small nativity set: Joseph, Mary and the baby Jesus. They were small enough to fit in the palm of my hand. I was filled with love for this man and his sweet wife. For perhaps the first time in my life, I knew the true spirit of Christmas.

We walked the Sussmans up front. There would be no fee this night. We wished them a Merry Christmas and saw them outside. It was snowing lightly, the first snowfall of the season. The flakes looked like powdered diamonds. I thought briefly of Grant and the dinner I had missed and knew that on this Christmas Eve, his grandmother would understand.

Carolyn S. Steele

Veronica's Babies

If someone listens, or stretches out a hand, or whispers a kind word of encouragement, or attempts to understand a lonely person, extraordinary things begin to happen.

Loretta Girzatlis

When I was in third grade, Mrs. Margaret McNeil was my teacher. She was young, vibrant and very pretty. She taught me and all the other impressionable boys and girls in her class the basics. Even those kids who were perceptually impaired or had serious disabilities miraculously learned, too. Everyone mastered third-grade reading and writing thanks to Mrs. McNeil—and Veronica.

Veronica was a huge, variegated spider plant suspended in the window of our classroom in a large, glistening-white, hanging basket. Every year, it produced babies—little plantlets on slender stems that cascaded over the rim of the pot. When you learned to read and write to Mrs. McNeil's "satisfaction," you were awarded one of Veronica's babies. None of the students could wait to get one.

On the big day, first you watered Veronica, and then Mrs. McNeil handed you the special scissors. You got to snip off a baby and name it. With Mrs. McNeil guiding you, you next planted it in moist soil in a styrofoam cup and wrote its new name on the outside with a green marker.

I'll never forget that March day when I had learned to read and write well enough. I went through Mrs. McNeil's ritual and carried home a small plant. I named it Rose, after my mother. I was so proud because I was one of the first boys to get one.

By the time June rolled around, every boy and girl in the class had received one of Veronica's babies. Even Billy Acker, who was mildly retarded and struggled the hardest of all of us, did well enough to get one.

Over the summer, we all had to promise to write Mrs. McNeil a letter and let her know how Veronica's baby was doing. She advised us to use a dictionary to help with difficult spellings.

I remember writing that my mom and dad helped me transplant the baby into a white hanging basket, and that its roots had grown really long.

During the summer, I kept my baby outside on our patio, and when fall arrived, I took it indoors to hang in front of my sliding glass door, where it got plenty of good light.

Years passed and Veronica's baby thrived. It produced babies, just as Veronica had done—many babies. I snipped them off and potted them up in hanging baskets, five to a basket. My dad would take them to work and sell them to his coworkers. With the extra money, I'd buy more hanging baskets and soil, and eventually I started a small business.

Thanks to Veronica's baby, I became interested in houseplants. Of course, my dad, who nurtured my interest in all kinds of plants, gets some of the credit, too. And while Mrs. McNeil first taught me to read and write well, it was Dad, again, who cultivated these skills in me.

When he called one weekend recently to tell me Mrs. McNeil had passed away, I knew I had to attend the wake. I journeyed home and sat with my wife, Carole, in a crowded funeral parlor. Mrs. McNeil lay there as if she were peacefully asleep. Her hair was silver, and there were many wrinkles on her powdered face, but other than that, she looked just as I remembered her. Hanging to her left by the window was Veronica, with many babies cascading over the rim of her basket. Veronica, unlike Mrs. McNeil, hadn't changed one bit.

Many people chatted about their remembrances of Mrs. McNeil, of third grade, of learning how to read and write better in order to get one of Veronica's babies, of her dedication.

When a vaguely familiar face rose to speak, the place grew suddenly silent.

"Hello, my name is Billy Acker," the man stammered. "Everyone told my mom and dad that I'd never be able to read and write because I was retarded. Ha! Mrs. McNeil taught me good how to read and write. She taught me real good."

He paused, and a large tear rolled down his cheek and stained the lapel of his gray suit. "You know, I still have one of Veronica's babies."

He wiped his eyes with the back of his hand and continued. "Every time I write or read an order in the shop, I can't help but think of Mrs. McNeil and how hard she worked with me after school. She taught me real good."

Many others spoke about Mrs. McNeil after Billy, but none matched him for his sincerity and simplicity.

Before we left, Carole and I talked to Mrs. McNeil's daughters and admired all the beautiful flower arrangements that lined the room. A good half of them were from

Acker's Florist. A huge, heart-shaped spray of white car-
nations with a bold red banner caught our attention at the
back of the room. Written in big black letters, it said: *If you
can read this, thank a teacher.* Underneath it, in shaky, almost
illegible penmanship, were the words: *Thank you Mrs.
McNeil. Love, your student, Billy Acker.*

George M. Flynn

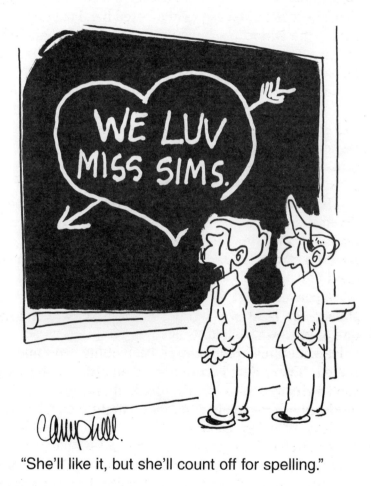

"She'll like it, but she'll count off for spelling."

Reprinted by permission of Martha Campbell.

Seeing with the Heart

Nothing in life is so hard that you can't make it easier by the way you take it.

Ellen Glasgow

I was blind! It was only for six weeks, but it seemed an eternity.

During that time, I was in a Columbus hospital, very scared, very alone, and extremely homesick for my husband and five kids. I am sure the darkness exaggerated these feelings even more. I spent hours, even days, wondering if I would ever be able to see my children again. I had spent so much time feeling sorry for myself that when the nurse announced I was getting a roommate, I was far from excited. Ironically, I didn't want anyone to "see" me this way. Like it or not, within a short time, my roommate moved into the bed on the other side of the room. Her name was Joni.

Despite my best efforts to dwell in self-pity, I almost immediately started liking Joni. She had such a positive attitude, was always so cheerful, and never complained about her own illness. She often sensed my fear and depression and somehow convinced me that I was lucky not to be able to see myself in the mirror during this time. My hair was a mess from lying in bed for a week, and I had gained several pounds from the cortisone IV's. Joni could always get me to laugh at her crazy jokes.

When Joe, my husband, came to visit, he sometimes brought all five kids with him. Can you imagine dressing five kids under six years old? It often took hours to find ten shoes and socks that matched. I had coded the kids' clothes in those days, and all you had to do was match a Pooh Bear top with a Pooh Bear bottom, and your child was in style! Well, Joe didn't know this, so the kids came to visit in quite a mixture of costumes. After they were gone, Joni spent hours telling me what each one had worn. Then she read to me all the little "I love you's" and "Please get well soon, Mommy's" from the cards they had brought. When friends sent fresh flowers, she described them to me. She opened my mail and told me how lucky I was to have so many friends. She helped me at mealtime to find my mouth with the food. Again, she convinced me that just for the moment perhaps, I was lucky that I couldn't see the hospital food!

One evening, Joe came alone. Joni must have sensed our need to be alone; she was so quiet I wasn't sure she was in the room. During his visit, Joe and I talked about the possibility that I might never see again. He assured me that nothing could change his love for me, and that somehow, no matter what, we would always have each other. Together we would continue to raise our family. For hours, he just held me in his arms, let me cry, and tried to make my dark world a tiny bit brighter.

After he left, I heard Joni stirring in her bed. When I asked her if she was awake, she said, "Don't you know how lucky you are to have so many people loving you? Your husband and kids are so beautiful! You are so lucky!"

At that moment, I realized for the first time that during our weeks together in the hospital, Joni hadn't had a husband or child visiting her. Her mother and minister came occasionally, but they only stayed a very short time.

I had been so wrapped up in myself, I hadn't even allowed her to confide in me. From her doctor's visits, I knew she was very sick, but I didn't even know with what. Once, I heard her doctor call her illness by a long Latin name, but I had never asked what it meant. I hadn't even taken the time to inquire. I realized how selfish I had become, and I hated myself for it. I turned over and started to cry. I asked God to forgive me. I promised the first thing the next morning, I would ask Joni about her illness, and I'd let her know how grateful I was to her for all she had done for me. I'd tell her that I did indeed love her.

I never got the chance. When I awoke the next morning, the curtain was pulled between our beds. I could hear people whispering nearby. I strained to hear what they were saying. Then I heard a minister repeating, "May she rest in eternal peace." Before I could tell her I loved her, Joni had died.

I learned later that Joni had come to the hospital for that very reason. She knew when she was admitted that she would never return home. Yet she had never complained and had spent the final days of her life giving hope to me.

Joni must have sensed her life was ending that last night when she told me how lucky I was. After I had cried myself to sleep, she had written me a note. The day nurse read it to me that morning, and when my vision later came back, I read it time and again:

My friend,

Thank you for making my last days so special! I found great happiness in our friendship. I know that you care for me, too, "sight unseen." Sometimes to get our full attention, God must knock us down, or at least make us blind. With my final breath, I pray that you will soon be seeing again, but not especially in the way you think. If you can only learn to see with your heart, then your life will be complete.

Remember me with love,
Joni

That night, I awoke from a deep sleep. As I lay in bed, I realized I could vaguely see the brightness of the tiny light along the baseboard. My vision was coming back! Only a little bit, but I could see!

Yet even more important, for the first time in my life, I could also see with my heart. Even though I never knew what Joni looked like, I am sure she was one of the most beautiful people in the world.

I have lost my vision several times since, but thanks to Joni, I will never allow myself to "lose sight" of the important things in life . . . things like warmth and love and sometimes even sorrow.

Barbara Jeanne Fisher

A Jelly Bean for Halloween

The bag of assorted candies was ready, and I'd been looking forward to visits from pint-sized goblins. But Halloween morning, my arthritis flared up, and by evening, I could barely move. I couldn't possibly answer each knock on the door to distribute the goodies, so I decided to fasten the candy bag to the door and watch the parade of trick-or-treaters from my darkened living room.

The first to arrive was a ballet dancer with three little ghosts. Each picked out a sweet in turn. When the last tiny hand emerged full-fisted, I heard the ballerina scold: "You're not supposed to take more than one!" I was pleased big sister would play conscience for the little one.

Princesses, astronauts, skeletons and aliens followed. More children showed up than I had expected. The candy was running low, and I was about to turn off the porch light when I noticed four more visitors. The three oldest reached into the bag and pulled out Hershey bars. I held my breath, hoping there would be one left for the tiny witch. But when she pulled out her hand, all it held was a single orange jelly bean.

Already the others were calling, "C'mon, Emily, let's

go. There's no one home to give you more." But Emily lingered an extra moment. She dropped the candy in her bag and then paused, facing the doors. Deliberately, she said, "Thank you, house. I like the jelly bean."

Then I watched her scamper away to join her fellow trick-or-treaters. One dear little witch had cast her spell on me.

Evelyn M. Gibb

THE FAMILY CIRCUS   By Bil Keane

"People who don't give me anything
get turned into a FROG!"

Reprinted by permission of Bil Keane.

Unexpected Angels

If I've learned anything on this crazy journey of mine, it's that around every bend in the road, and at the end of even the darkest tunnel, there's likely to be a company of angels.

With me, though, they're more likely to be Hell's Angels!

A few years ago my husband, Karl, and son, J. J., and I were in our van, traveling through Massachusetts to visit my cousins. It was very late, about two or three in the morning, when it became clear that we were lost. The country roads seemed to be going on forever, and the farther we traveled, the worse it seemed to get.

Finally we came upon one of those big granddaddy truck stops. So we pulled in for directions. Karl was really shot from all the driving, so I got out of the van to do the talking.

"Does anybody here know how to find Merridale Road?" I asked.

A very tired waitress looked up and said, "Lady, I haven't got a clue."

Since she was not going to be any help, I looked around at the customers. There, sitting nearby, were four of the toughest human beings I had ever seen in my life. Chains. Black leather. Skulls and crossbones. The whole bit.

I immediately thought of my family in the van and what these characters might do to us.

"We know where you're going," one of them said cheerfully. "Not only that, but we'll take you there."

Before I could say no, they got up off their chairs, paid their bill, and were outside on their motorcycles, gesturing, "Follow us!"

We started to follow this large motorcycle gang down lonely Massachusetts country roads in the wee hours of the morning. There were four guys on motorcycles and four women who weighed 300 pounds each sitting behind them.

After a few minutes, J. J. decided it was all over for us. "They're taking us to a lonely spot, and that will be the end," he said ominously. "I'm never going to see my school or my friends again. How could you do this to me?"

I whispered to Karl, "I don't want to scare J. J., but he's right. I am a bit frightened. It's dark. The road is getting very lonely. And these people are tough. Maybe I did the wrong thing."

"No kidding," he retorted. "We're just going to have to trust that it's going to be all right."

"If they tell us to stop," I said, "don't stop. Gun the motor and keep going."

About an hour later, after winding through endless back roads deep in the woods, they motioned to us to go left.

We looked up, and there was the sign for Merridale Road. They had put us on the right road after all.

As they waved good-bye, I heard someone shout, "Keep up the good work, Sally!"

They had known who I was all along, yet they had never let on.

About six months later, when Burt was finishing the warmup for the television show, I looked out in the studio audience and thought I saw an apparition.

There, sitting right smack in front of a bunch of proper Connecticut housewives, was the same motorcycle gang.

Burt took one look at the unsavory foursome and said aghast, "Do you see those people? What are we going to do?"

"Not only do I see them," I said, "but I know them." With that I took the mike and went over and renewed our friendship.

Ever since then, whenever I see or read anything about the Hell's Angels, I get a smile on my lips.

I remember how they once led me down the road—the long, unknown road to adventure. And how, at the end, I was treated to the biggest surprise of all.

Sally Jessy Raphaël

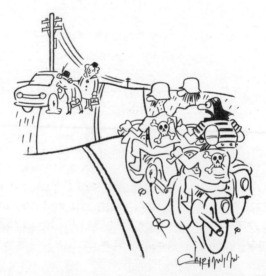

"Think they'd panic if we stopped to help?"

Beauty Contest

A successful beauty product company asked the people in a large city to send brief letters about the most beautiful women they knew, along with the women's pictures. Within a few weeks, thousands of letters were delivered to the company.

One letter in particular caught the attention of the employees, and soon it was handed to the company president. The letter was written by a young boy, who wrote he was from a broken home, living in a run-down neighborhood. With spelling corrections, an excerpt from his letter read:

> A beautiful woman lives down the street from me. I visit her every day. She makes me feel like the most important kid in the world. We play checkers and she listens to my problems. She understands me and when I leave, she always yells out the door that she's proud of me.

The boy ended his letter by saying, "This picture shows you that she is the most beautiful woman. I hope I have a wife as pretty as her."

Intrigued by the letter, the president asked to see this woman's picture. His secretary handed him a photograph of a smiling, toothless woman, well-advanced in years, sitting in a wheelchair. Sparse gray hair was pulled back in a bun and wrinkles that formed deep furrows on her face were somehow diminished by the twinkle in her eyes.

"We can't use this woman," explained the president, smiling. "She would show the world that our products aren't necessary to be beautiful."

Carla Muir

The Scar

His thumb softly rubbed the twisted flesh on my cheek. The plastic surgeon, a good fifteen years my senior, was a very attractive man. His masculinity and the intensity of his gaze seemed almost overpowering.

"Hmmm," he said quietly. "Are you a model?"

Is this a joke? Is he kidding? I asked myself, and I searched his handsome face for signs of mockery. No way would anyone ever confuse me with a fashion model. I was ugly. My mother casually referred to my sister as her pretty child. Anyone could see I was homely. After all, I had the scar to prove it.

The accident happened in fourth grade, when a neighbor boy picked up a hunk of concrete and heaved the mass through the side of my face. An emergency room doctor stitched together the shreds of skin, pulling catgut through the tattered outside of my face and then suturing the shards of flesh inside my mouth. For the rest of the year, a huge bandage from cheekbone to jaw covered the raised angry welt.

A few weeks after the accident, an eye exam revealed I was nearsighted. Above the ungainly bandage sat a big, thick pair of glasses. Around my head, a short fuzzy glob of curls stood out like mold growing on old bread. To save money, Mom had taken me to a beauty school where a student cut my hair. The overzealous girl hacked away cheerfully. Globs of hair piled up on the floor. By the time her instructor wandered over, the damage was done. A quick conference followed, and we were given a coupon for a free styling on our next visit.

"Well," sighed my father that evening, "you'll always be pretty to me," and he hesitated, "even if you aren't to the rest of the world."

Right. Thanks. As if I couldn't hear the taunts of the other kids at school. As if I couldn't see how different I looked from the little girls whom the teachers fawned over. As if I didn't occasionally catch a glimpse of myself in the bathroom mirror. In a culture that values beauty, an ugly girl is an outcast. My looks caused me no end of pain. I sat in my room and sobbed every time my family watched a beauty pageant or a "talent" search show.

Eventually I decided that if I couldn't be pretty, I would at least be well-groomed. Over the course of years, I learned to style my hair, wear contact lenses and apply make-up. Watching what worked for other women, I learned to dress myself to best advantage. And now, I was engaged to be married. The scar, shrunken and faded with age, stood between me and a new life.

"Of course, I'm not a model," I replied with a small amount of indignation.

The plastic surgeon crossed his arms over his chest and looked at me appraisingly. "Then why are you concerned about this scar? If there is no professional reason to have it removed, what brought you here today?"

Suddenly he represented all the men I'd ever known. The eight boys who turned me down when I invited them to the girls-ask-boys dance. The sporadic dates I'd had in college. The parade of men who had ignored me since then. The man whose ring I wore on my left hand. My hand rose to my face. The scar confirmed it; I was ugly. The room swam before me as my eyes filled with tears.

The doctor pulled a rolling stool up next to me and sat down. His knees almost touched mine. His voice was low and soft.

"Let me tell you what I see. I see a beautiful woman. Not a perfect woman, but a beautiful woman. Lauren Hutton has a gap between her front teeth. Elizabeth Taylor has a tiny, tiny scar on her forehead," he almost whispered. Then he paused and handed me a mirror. "I think to myself how every remarkable woman has an imperfection, and I believe that imperfection makes her beauty more remarkable because it assures us she is human."

He pushed back the stool and stood up. "I won't touch it. Don't let anyone fool with your face. You are delightful just the way you are. Beauty really does come from within a woman. Believe me. It is my business to know."

Then he left.

I turned to the face in the mirror. He was right. Somehow over the years, that ugly child had become a beautiful woman. Since that day in his office, as a woman who makes her living speaking before hundreds of people, I have been told many times by people of both sexes that I am beautiful. And, I know I am.

When I changed how I saw myself, others were forced to change how they saw me. The doctor didn't remove the scar on my face; he removed the scar on my heart.

Joanna Slan

The Melding

Your task is not to seek for love, but merely to seek and find all the barriers within yourself that you have built against it.

Rumi

My husband and I came from different religious backgrounds—mine Christian, his Jewish—and moreover, we were both fiery and determined individuals. Consequently, our first few years together tested our ability to respect and combine our two religious traditions with love and understanding. I remember raising the subject of a Christmas tree the first December after our marriage.

"Christmas tree?" LeRoy exclaimed incredulously. "Listen, there are two things I won't do. Buying a ham is one of them. Buying a Christmas tree is the other."

"If I can grate my knuckles while making potato latkes and clean up drippy candles at Chanukah, you can suffer through a Christmas tree!" I snapped back.

"No way," he retorted. "Remember last month? Whom do I meet at the grocery store when I have nothing but a ham in my cart? The rabbi. If we went shopping for a

Christmas tree together, the whole synagogue would probably pass by on a bus while I was loading it into the trunk! Forget it!"

Naturally, we got a tree. A big, beautiful, feathery spruce that claimed half the living room in our tiny apartment. Or, as LeRoy scornfully referred to it in front of our Jewish friends, a "moldy-green matzo ball with colored lights." However, despite LeRoy's professed antagonism, when Christmas morning arrived, I noticed that the number of gifts beneath the tree had doubled—and the tags they bore were written in LeRoy's hand.

By the time our daughter Erica was born, we had faced and solved many of the problems of an interfaith marriage and agreed to combine our heritages in an effort to provide the best for our children. By the time Shauna arrived three years later, we had settled into a way of life that was comfortable for both of us, although a bit unusual. Holly around the menorah. Chicken soup, matzo balls with oregano, and potato latkes for Christmas dinner. Merry Chanukah. Fa-la-la-la. Happy Christmas. Shalom. We were discovering that peace means the same in any language.

At holiday time, our home was decorated with a potpourri of blue-and-white streamers, menorah lights, Advent calendars and a crèche. Our friends from both traditions joined in the spirit. A Christian neighbor brought us a glass mobile made of multiple Stars of David from the Holy Land. Our Jewish friends made and gave us many ornaments for the tree.

I became adept at reciting Hebrew prayers and explained Chanukah to both girls' classes every year. When LeRoy bought me a beautiful homemade guitar one Christmas, the first thing I taught myself to play and sing was a Jewish folk song. Dressed in a blue velvet shirt with buttons from Israel and a matching yarmulke (the skullcap worn by Jewish men at religious functions) that I had made him, LeRoy learned to warble off-key versions of the better-known carols.

One year, my husband brought home a little blue wooden Star of David. "This is for *your* tree," he stated crisply. "I want it to be the first ornament hung every year."

"I'll see to it personally, General," I quickly assured him, and from then on, it adorned the top of our tree.

One disconcerted Christian friend asked me, "Don't you feel hypocritical placing a Star of David on the top of your Christmas tree?"

"No," I replied and meant it. "Jesus was Jewish. And there was a star shining high over a stable. Remember?"

By this time, Chanukah had become almost as much a symbol of freedom and light to me as Christmas. And Christmas had become increasingly meaningful as the birthday of one so special that he gave light and freedom to everyone. As people of all races and religions gathered in our home, we found that their differences enriched our lives. The holidays seemed to become even more joyous.

Then, not long after we had celebrated our eleventh wedding anniversary, my forty-two-year-old husband suffered three heart attacks within two months. On December 17, our daughters and I crowded onto his narrow hospital bed in the intensive care unit to sing Chanukah and Christmas songs. The next night, the first night of Chanukah, I was driving to a friend's house where Erica and Shauna would kindle the first Chanukah lights. Suddenly, in my mind, I saw a dazzling burst of light, and then the image of a smiling, healthy LeRoy. When we reached our friend's house, I learned that at sundown, LeRoy had leaned over and whispered, "Shalom, shalom" to his rabbi, who was seated by his hospital bed. Then LeRoy's soul had departed this earth.

The following evening, friends and relatives arrived at our home to sit shivah, the Jewish period of mourning.

In the lights provided by the silver menorah's candles and the twinkling Christmas tree, Jewish men in yarmulkes and prayer shawls bowed their heads and opened worn copies of the Old Testament. The doorbell rang. I opened the door and found members of Erica's fourth-grade class assembled there. As they began to sing "Silent Night," my daughters rushed to stand beside me in the doorway. I gathered Shauna and Erica into my arms. Behind us, we could hear the comforting Hebrew words chanted by men LeRoy had loved. In front of us, Erica's schoolmates sang the ancient carol in their clear, childish voices. The love radiating from these two traditions gave sudden, special meaning to LeRoy's and my marriage. In that one moment, my grief fell away, and I felt LeRoy's presence.

"Shalom, my love," I whispered.

"Sleep in heavenly peace," the children sang sweetly and triumphantly.

"Daddy's with God now, isn't he?" Shauna asked.

"Yes," I told her firmly. "Whatever road he took to get there, he's certainly with God."

Twenty Chanukahs and twenty Christmases have come and gone since that night, but the love that fused our hearts and lives remains vibrant in our home. Every December, the prayers of Chanukah as well as of Christmas still echo through the house, and the green holly encircles the silver menorah on the windowsill. The little blue Star of David still takes its lofty place as the first ornament placed on the Christmas tree, shining from on high—as did the star above that stable in Bethlehem so long ago—to proclaim peace on earth, goodwill to men.

Isabel Bearman Bucher

Old People

At age ninety-two, Grandma Fritz still lived in her old two-story farmhouse, made homemade noodles, and did her laundry in her wringer-washer in the basement. She maintained her vegetable garden, big enough to feed all of Benton County, with just a hoe and spade. Her seventy-year-old children lovingly protested when she insisted on mowing her huge lawn with her ancient push mower.

"I only work outside in the cool, early mornings and in the evenings," Grandma explained, "and I always wear my sunbonnet."

Still, her children were understandably relieved when they heard she was attending the noon lunches at the local senior citizens' center.

Yes, Grandma admitted, as her daughter nodded approvingly. "I cook for them. Those old people appreciate it so much!"

LeAnn Thieman

3

LIVE YOUR DREAMS

You are never given a dream without also being given the power to make it true.

Richard Bach

A Star to Steer By

If you seek what is honorable, what is good, what is the truth of your life, all the other things you could not imagine come as a matter of course.

Oprah Winfrey

Anybody can become a widow. There aren't any special qualifications. It happens in less time than it takes to draw a breath. It doesn't require the planning, for example, that it takes to become a wife or a mother or any of the other ritual roles of womanhood. And it is neither dramatic nor majestic—really more a snapshot than a feature film. For such a monumental thing to be accomplished in seconds defies logic—in fact, it's almost insulting. But there it is.

My husband, Dan, died of cancer on a sunny June morning, when the grip of a Wisconsin winter had finally relaxed and the very air was a bath on the skin. It was the last day of school, and I'd assured my two middle sons, then in first and third grades, that nothing could happen to Daddy in the one hour it would take to pick up their report cards. Our teenager was getting ready for her senior prom; the littlest, just turned four, was downstairs with Michelle, our caregiver.

I was looking forward to an hour's sleep.

All night, I'd napped on the floor near our bed with my friend Jean Marie, a nurse. Between Dan's low moans and the *thump-hiss* of the oxygen tank, we'd managed little rest. So, newly showered and wearing my aged flannel nightgown—the one Dan used to call my "don't even ask" nightgown—I lay down beside my husband of thirteen years, my editor and my buddy for most of my adult life.

I don't believe in signs and portents. But I've come to think that the atmosphere in a room does take on the coloration of a significant change. For some reason, I leaned close to Dan's ear as he breathed in, and then, thirty seconds later, slowly out, and I whispered, "You are the best-smelling man. You are the sexiest man. It's been a privilege to be married to you." Dan gave a kind of hiccup. Then he was dead. He had just turned forty-five; I was forty.

You imagine that your tears, so long suppressed, will flood from you and your wails shake the walls.

Yet, I merely sat down next to this body, which had been as familiar to me as my own and was no less so now, and let my fingers trace the line of his nose—already, amazingly, cooling.

The front door banged open, and my sons rushed in from school. Michelle called up for me to sign for a package. I put on my jeans and washed Dan's face with the hem of my old nightgown, promising myself I would never wear it again, though in fact I wear it all the time. If I could only manage to see all this as terribly sad instead of crippling and horrifying, I remember instructing myself, I would not break in half. The worse moment, after all, had come four months before, when Dan—who went into the hospital with a little digestive disturbance—was diagnosed overnight with end-stage, do-not-pass-go colon cancer, for which any kind of therapy would be just an exercise. My husband, a small-town newspaper editor, had been a stand-up guy in life, in print and in death. All he said, when he heard the worst, was, "My babies, my babies."

Now mine, alone.

That thought kept me upright as I gathered our children to his bedside, and later, when I told hundreds of his assembled colleagues and friends, "It's tempting, when something like this happens to someone so young, to say that life's a bitch and then you die. But to do that would dishonor the very reason this is all so sad—which is that life is wonderful, and most wonderful for its smallest splendors: good coffee, children who smell like rain, bickering about whether to fix the linoleum."

Dan's suffering was over, but I'd somehow forgotten, in the years of our marriage, to observe the line where his life left off and mine began. I felt lame, stupid, at a distance from myself. As for the children, who live in time differently from adults, each day was not a step toward healing, but another step away from Dan. Through my wall at night, I could hear my eldest son sobbing, "Daddy, please, please." We commenced the months of undone schoolwork, visits to counselors, fights on the playground. My four-year-old came home one day with a tight and secret smile. "Mike's a big baby," he said. "He thinks you can wish on a star, and it will come real. I know it won't come real, because I wished on a star for ten nights. And it's just a big story."

Meanwhile, the roof, quite literally, fell in. That, and all manner of other bewildering debts and choices loomed. I'd been working part-time in the public relations department of a university and trying to realize the dream of supporting myself with my writing. Dan had encouraged it, but I'd counted on his support. Now I had to figure out how to regroup.

Get rid of your sitter, friends said. *The kids have to learn there's no money for such things. Get a smaller house. And a steady job.* My well-intentioned father recommended speaking to a friend about a public relations position at a machine factory that made ball bearings. "You can't take chances anymore," he said. "Playtime is over. They'll always need ball bearings."

Working at least part of the week in my little office while my youngest played upstairs, I tried to put off giving up the way of life I loved. I wrote feverishly, often with two of my best friends at my elbow, helping me when I forgot the past tense of common verbs. Editors I'd never met scrambled generously to throw work my way.

But I knew that I was only treading water. One night, after paying the plumber, I was down to $86. The kids' education fund had long been spent, mostly on home repairs, and I knew that even when Dan's life insurance came through, it wouldn't tide us over for long. It was time to fish or cut bait; past time. I needed to take my hat in hand and plead with the university or with the newspaper where I'd worked for years before that—or even with Mr. Ball Bearings—to give me reliable full-time work.

It was a good thing.

It was the right thing.

If it seemed somehow . . . smaller than the life I'd worked so hard to try to craft for myself, gradually burnishing my reputation as a freelance writer, cherishing the dream of spinning tales for fun and profit one day, at least it was safer. At least. My job now was salvage, not discovery. That's what everyone said.

I had lunch early that first spring after Dan's death with a close friend, an acclaimed novelist on the verge of publishing her breakthrough bestseller. We talked about the giddiness of her success, and then about rocks and hard places. I knew what I needed to do, I told Jane, so why did knowing that make me feel that I, too, was dying? As she indulgently drew me out, I told her something I'd told few other people—a story. I'd somehow dreamed it in its entirety one night before Dan became ill, though I'm not much of a narrative dreamer. It was about a big Italian family caught in an extraordinary crisis over their child. I knew their names, how they looked and what they would do. Given the way my life had turned out, I told Jane it was almost a relief to know I'd never have to find out that I couldn't write it. I wanted her to feel as sorry for me as I felt for myself. But instead she said, "Apply for a fellowship."

And study classical ballet, I agreed. And learn to spot-weld.

Hadn't I just explained in detail why almost everyone I knew expected me to downsize my dreams, not spin even more impractical plans? But she said, "Those are really good excuses. You should still do it."

I'm a practical woman. I wasn't convinced. But not long after, sitting on my porch in the middle of the night, mentally balancing columns of things I needed against things I could afford, I remembered something Dan had told me not long before he died. I'd been wailing about how I couldn't live without him, when he suddenly said to me, "Listen. In two years' time, you'll be far from here. You'll be a writer of merit. But you have to believe in it, like I believe in you."

Telling no one, I wrote for applications forms to The Ragdale Foundation in Lake Forest, Illinois, a competitive artists' program. I was accepted. Loading my scribbled notes, a thesaurus, a Bible and a copy of *Wuthering Heights* into the back of the truck with my computer, I set out in October.

It should have been bliss, the first eight hours of solitude I could remember in my adult life. But I was a basket case. I talked a good act, but who knew if I could really write? Here I was, depriving my lonely children of my healing presence, and myself of three weeks' work, and for what? I locked the door of my beautiful room and cried.

The next morning, and for three weeks after, I wrote. During those three weeks, my daughter told me she was about to lose her scholarship, my older son went AWOL on a city bus for four hours while Michelle frantically searched for him, and my youngest cried nightly on the phone, but I wrote. Creditors phoned. Teachers were dismayed. Even my father thundered, "These *children* are your future, Jackie!" Still, I wrote. I was beginning to see this as my critical passage; there was nothing more to lose. If I didn't give it my best, my family's sacrifice would be meaningless.

And it was during this time that I really grieved Dan, and let my grief have life in the keening of another mother, Beth, a character in my book who'd lost even more than I had. I recalled all the agony of the past year, of the night in a therapist's office when my oldest son, Robert, told me, "You said Dad wouldn't die before I got home! I never got to say good-bye, and I hate your guts forever!" I unraveled that pain and reknit it, trying to be forgiven.

Six weeks after I came home, my agent sold my seventy-five pages to the publisher of her choice. Emboldened, I took a leave from the university to write the rest. I called my brother to tell him I'd decided to resign from my job and go it on my own.

"No," he said, horrified. "No, don't. Maybe three books from now. Don't do this. Think of the kids."

"I am," I said, with more conviction than I felt. "If I didn't do this, it wouldn't be showing much confidence in myself, would it?"

"There's such a thing," he said softly, "as too much confidence."

But last winter, when the book was optioned for a film, my brother celebrated: "This is like the TV movie where the team with the fat kid gets the trophy. You deserve to win!"

Happily ever after? Well, I work harder than I ever knew I could, and my children get angry when they have to give of my time in ways they would rather not. When they're hurt, I'm wretched. But none of us doubts that this is sacrifice in the service of something worthwhile.

Like most women in midlife, I got the same message from almost everyone: The key to maturity is to risk less and settle more. Even those who didn't intend to discourage me made it clear that, in my shoes, they would be more cautious, more conservative. To them, I must have seemed a woman thinking of herself instead of her responsibilities. But to me, making decisions based on fear felt lonely and humbling, not virtuous. Does a good mother teach her children to be timid, to trade down their dreams? Does she teach them that loss has to break our will even as it breaks our hearts?

And what is living—in the time we're given to do it— except daring?

One night, a neighbor took my children on a picnic so I could chip away at the mountain of final revisions on my book. I didn't expect to make an end that hot night, but suddenly, I was closing in on final words, and then, I was done. I wandered out to the porch with my coffee cup, and the night air was a warm bath on my skin. I'm sure I knew it on some level, but until that moment I didn't recognize it. It was June 4, 1995. Exactly two years to the day that Dan died.

I don't believe in signs and portents. And I don't believe there is any more in store for us than this life. On the other hand, my life has made me willing to be surprised. And so perhaps, someday, when the atmosphere in the room changes again and this time the knock is for me, I'll find out it was Dan, after all, blowing those beautiful fates in my direction.

That aside, there is a thing I do believe: I believe in the afterglow of a good and long relationship, like the light of a star that keeps pulsing visibly to Earth long after the star itself has been extinguished. It may not make your wishes come true, but it can light your way.

Jacquelyn Mitchard

[EDITORS' NOTE: *The book Jacquelyn dreamed,* The Deep End of the Ocean, *became a #1* New York Times *bestseller and was the first book Oprah Winfrey used to launch her Book-of-the-Month Club.*]

There She Is, Miss America

Dreams are renewable. No matter what our age or condition, there are still untapped possibilities within us and new beauty waiting to be born.

Dale Turner

September 17, 1994. My lack of nervousness had begun to make me nervous. The relaxed sense of peace I felt seemed such a contrast to the tension and excitement I'd experienced during all the other pageants in which my daughter, Heather, had competed. Yet this was Atlantic City—and the final night of the Miss America pageant. Tonight would bring either the remarkable culmination, or the sudden and disappointing end, of my daughter's incredible dream. Yet, the most pervasive sensation I'd had all evening was this disconcerting, yet clearly God-given, feeling of inner calm.

I hadn't worried at all about the evening gown competition; Heather had been elegant. She looked great and walked beautifully during the swimsuit segment as well. Then she'd justified my lack of jitters during the talent portion of the competition by captivating the entire audience with her electrifying performance—a classic ballet interpretation of Sandi Patty's inspirational song, "Via Dolorosa."

When Miss America's television hosts, Regis Philbin and Kathie Lee Gifford, announced the five finalists, the second name called was "Heather Whitestone, Miss Alabama." As the five finalists moved toward center stage, my maternal anxiety began to build.

All five contestants looked stunning. As a burst of orchestra music signaled the end of the commercial break, a hush of anticipation settled across that vast convention hall. My nightlong calm evaporated as the last notes of music faded away.

Twenty years ago this very night, eighteen-month-old Heather had lain critically ill in the pediatric ward of a hospital in Dothan, Alabama, while her doctors tried to decide what was wrong and how to treat her. Unbeknownst to us, sometime during her stay in the hospital, Heather had slipped into a world of silence.

Was it possible for my deaf child to find success and happiness in the hearing world? Sometimes I'd felt very alone in my belief that she could—or even should try. Most experts told us not to expect her to attain more than a third-grade education. And why even bother enrolling a deaf child in dance? While most people considered only Heather's limitations, fortunately, a few saw her potential.

Heather had worked long and hard to be here tonight. She hoped to become the first deaf Miss America—and be a bridge between the hearing and deaf worlds. Now I worried: Could a deaf girl who dreamed of becoming Miss America actually win the crown?

All this and more raced through my mind during the commercial break and then during Regis and Kathie Lee's time-killing chat with Miss America 1994, Kimberly Aiken.

Finally, the scores were tallied and the judges' decision delivered.

The envelope was opened, and Regis Philbin called out, "Fourth runner-up: Miss Indiana, Tiffany Storm." The crowd cheered, and my blood pressure jumped a few more points. "Third runner-up: Miss Georgia, Andrea Krahn." The three remaining contestants stood at center stage holding hands. "Second runner-up: Miss New Jersey, Jennifer Alexis Makris."

As the cheering subsided, Regis went on to say, "Here we are now. Down to two. That leaves Miss Alabama and Miss Virginia."

Kathie Lee now said, "One of you beautiful ladies will win a $20,000 scholarship to continue your education, and the other will win a $35,000 scholarship, plus the crown and the title of Miss America."

"Okay," said Regis. "This is it, everybody! Ladies and gentlemen, the winner of a $20,000 scholarship is . . . Miss Virginia, Cullen Johnson. And the new Miss America 1995: Miss Alabama, Heather Whitestone!"

The crowd of 13,000 packing the Atlantic City Convention Center exploded into wall-shaking cheers. The bewildered expression on Heather's face told me she hadn't understood the announcement. It wasn't until Cullen pointed at her, mouthed the words, "It's you!" and gave her a big congratulatory hug that Heather realized she'd won.

I never did clearly see what happened next. I could tell Heather was crying. I was crying. My mother and sisters were crying. Stacey and Melissa, Heather's two older sisters, were screaming and jumping up and down. All of Heather's cousins and her aunts and uncles were cheering and applauding like mad. My father, in joyous celebration of Heather's victory, was punching his arms into the air and screaming, "YES! YES! YES!"

I guess Regis and Kathie Lee must have been singing, "There she is, Miss America . . . " because Heather was now walking down the runway and waving to the crowd. But all that our family and friends could hear was the sound of wild cheering, our own and everyone else's around us.

When Heather made her turn and strolled back toward the stage, I could see her searching for the family in the crowd. I don't know why she didn't spot us immediately: We were the contingent of fools screaming and jumping up and down. There were thirty of us wildly waving and flashing her the familiar hand sign for "I love you." When she finally spotted us, she signed her love back to us, and we all screamed even louder.

My heart was so full. She'd done it! Heather had dreamed of this day for so long. As hard and impossible as it had seemed at times for someone deaf to become Miss America, tonight I was ecstatic that I had always told her, "Yes, you can, Heather! Yes—you can!"

Daphne Gray

Born to Sing

The girl seemed born to sing. She had such a perfect sense of pitch that in her later years, she could tell when one player out of an entire orchestra played a wrong note. She never took singing lessons and she never learned to read music—she learned "by ear."

At the age of fourteen, the young girl developed gland trouble, which caused her to gain weight. As she continued to gain, the children at school began to tease her. Upset, she would hurry home from school, shut herself in her room and cry. This pattern continued and her family worried about her spending so much time alone. Her grandmother urged her to forget about her weight and to concentrate on developing her lovely voice.

She took her grandmother's advice, and before long she was winning prizes at the amateur nights put on by the local theater. More than anything else, the girl wanted to become a professional singer, but her parents thought it would be better if she studied nursing. They thought her enormous size might be too much of a handicap for a successful stage career.

She started nurses' training, but she longed to be

singing instead. Finally, she decided to give up nursing and pursue her dreams. In her heart, she believed that people would forget her looks when they heard her voice.

She went to Broadway and soon she got a small part in a musical comedy. She was thrilled with the opportunity to sing, but she was cast with a man whose part called for him to make jokes about her weight.

The jokes brought down the house with laughter. The young woman was deeply hurt inside, but she refused to give up. She had signed a contract and so she stayed with the show through its run on Broadway.

One night, she received a note backstage saying that a man would like to see her. At first she was afraid it might be one of those jokers who delighted in taking her to a fancy restaurant, urging her to eat a great deal, and then laughing with his friends about it later.

But the man who wanted to see her that night changed her life.

He was Ted Collins, of the Columbia Record Company. He became her manager and lifelong friend, encouraging and guiding her through the many happy years of her subsequent singing career.

First, she made records for Columbia. Later, her big opportunity came when she was asked to broadcast a radio show. Soon, the whole country was singing her theme song, "When the Moon Comes Over the Mountain." And it was her rendition of "God Bless America" that made it America's "second national anthem."

By 1940, she was topping all the radio polls in the country. When television came, she was offered the chance to have her own show. But on television she would be seen by millions of people. She thought of the early days, when audiences had laughed at her because she was so fat. Why should she take a chance that it might happen again? She didn't need the money—radio had made her both wealthy and famous.

It was her tremendous love of singing that gave her courage and she decided to take the risk. Almost at once her rich voice won her the admiration of television audiences, and a new generation began humming, "When the Moon Comes Over the Mountain."

Eventually, because she radiated such warmth, sincerity and charm, she became a symbol of the things people love about our country—generosity, kindness and good will towards all people.

It was no wonder that when President Franklin D. Roosevelt introduced her to King George and Queen Elizabeth, he said:

"This is Kate Smith. This is America."

Ravina Gelfand and Letha Patterson
Submitted by Oscar H. Greene

Truly Free

Hold fast to dreams for if dreams die, life is a broken-winged bird that cannot fly.

Langston Hughes

Life was hard in Cuba. In the early 1980s, hundreds of Cubans tried to reach United States soil aboard makeshift rafts. Some made the trip successfully and were allowed to settle in America. But many more were not so lucky and were stopped and arrested before they could escape—or worse, they became victims of the sea. It is a long ninety miles from Cuba to Key West when your ship is an old tire.

One young woman, named Margherita, was persistent in her determination to break free. Margherita's ambition was to practice medicine. She knew this dream could never become a reality in her Communist homeland, because most Cubans who hold medical degrees end up making better livings driving taxis. The rest of her family had all made it to the United States, leaving her alone in a country where she had little hope of a better life.

Margherita tried to escape on several different occasions, but always failed. She was a strong-willed woman, not a desirable trait in this Communist society. Soon, government officials began harassing her on a routine basis. She was often awakened in the middle of the night by police who were sent to check upon her whereabouts. She was discovered during one escape attempt and promptly arrested before she ever put her raft into the water.

As a result, Margherita was fired from her job in the tourism sector and forced to wash dishes for a period of one year, without pay. Often, police—who insisted upon checking her identification card—stopped her in the streets. There was no peace in her life, and her dream was slowly dying. Finally, the repercussions of her failed escape became too much for her to handle. She contemplated suicide.

But Margherita had too much spirit, too much hope, to take her own life. She decided to plan another escape, but this time, she enlisted two others to help her. She and her accomplices pooled their resources and bought an old truck inner tube, wood and some rope. On the appointed day, they met after midnight and managed to set themselves afloat, praying for a safe journey to freedom. But not far from shore, Margherita and her friends met with serious trouble. Not with the government, but with Mother Nature.

There were storms in the ocean, and their tiny craft was severely tested. They weathered the wind and rain for two days, and floated aimlessly for another. The three were severely dehydrated and beaten cruelly by the waves before being rescued by the U.S. Coast Guard. They had traveled seventy-seven miles during their four-day journey. They were allowed into the country, where Margherita was quickly reunited with her family.

Margherita was free! She enrolled in college and began to work toward her goal of being a doctor. Although her studies were demanding, they were a welcome challenge.

Margherita spent many nights reading until the early hours of the morning, but she was happy to do it.

About a year later, she was up late studying for a final exam. Resting her eyes for a moment, she sat quietly, remembering how life had been for her in Cuba. She felt her chest tighten as she recalled all her misery. Life had felt like a dead-end there, and worse, she had been treated with disrespect and cruelty. She felt her anger begin to rise as she thought of the injustices she had endured. She remembered the harassment she received from the Cuban officials—and from one man in particular. Although it was nearly two in the morning, she decided to call this official at his home in Cuba. She had called him so often when he had been her probation officer that she still remembered his phone number. *I will wake him up from his sound sleep. I'll give him a taste of his own medicine and see how he likes it,* she thought.

Margherita did not allow herself time for a change of heart, but quickly dialed his number. She grew angrier, stewing in her unpleasant memories as she awaited the connection of the phone line.

When the Cuban official answered his telephone, she did not hesitate to speak. "It is me, Margherita, the young woman you harassed all those months. I am calling to thank you," she said.

"To thank me?" he asked, surprised.

"Yes. I am now a medical student in the United States. It was your endless harassment that made my life unbearable in Cuba. You forced me to come to this rich country where a woman can make her dreams come true," she explained, her voice triumphant with this small revenge.

She was surprised when the Cuban official let out a deep sigh. He was silent for a few moments, then said, "My own life here is very difficult. I must watch my daughter dying, a little each day, from a liver illness. The only advice I get from the doctors is to give her six aspirin a day—" At that point his voice began to break.

"You called to wake me, to repay me for my harassment, to make me suffer. But I tell you, I am already suffering as I stay awake each long night, trying to comfort my poor little girl. She is losing her life to this sickness because I do not have enough money to buy aspirin. And even if I did, there would be no aspirin available to me."

The man was now sobbing into the phone, broken with grief. Shocked, Margherita did not know how to respond. In a daze, she mumbled her regrets into the phone and then hung up. She sat for a long time, staring at her books without seeing them.

It is only what he deserves, she told herself. *He made my life miserable.* But she could no longer find her anger, her fiery ambition. Something completely different filled her heart.

The next morning, Margherita hurried to the pharmacy. She bought as much aspirin as she could afford, packed it in a big box and sent it—with love—to her old enemy, the government official in Cuba. *Now,* she thought, *I am truly free.*

Elizabeth Bravo

You Can Do It!

Just don't give up trying to do what you really want to do. Where there's love and inspiration, I don't think you can go wrong.

Ella Fitzgerald

The confidence my mother instilled in me has served me throughout my adult life. Without it, Mary Kay Inc. might have fizzled before it even began. It was 1963. After twenty-five years as a professional saleswoman, with my children grown, I just decided that retirement did not suit me. And so I had developed a strategy and philosophy for beginning my own "dream company." I had recruited several salespeople and invested my life savings in the chance of a lifetime. Using my years of experience in direct sales, I was going to train and supervise the Beauty Consultants, while my husband was going to handle the administrative details of our new business. We had assembled boxes of bottles and jars and brand-new labels that read, "Beauty by Mary Kay."

Exactly one month before we were scheduled to open, my husband and I were having breakfast together. He was reading the final percentage figures for our company, and I was listening very much as a wife often does when her husband talks about the budget—with half an ear, because I considered it to be "his problem." At that moment, he suffered a fatal heart attack.

I believe that work is often the best antidote for grief. And so, despite my shock, I decided to open the business as planned. Starting the company had been my dream and my idea, but I had never imagined that I would run it alone. I knew that I didn't have the needed administrative skills; and yet, at this point, all the merchandise, bottles and labels were useless if the company folded. I *had* to go on.

I turned to both my attorney and my accountant for advice.

"Mary Kay," my attorney said, shaking his head, "liquidate the business right now and recoup whatever cash you can. If you don't, you'll end up penniless."

I had hoped that my accountant would be a little more encouraging, but after studying the situation he said, "You can't possibly do it. This commission schedule will never work. It's just a matter of time before the company goes bankrupt—and you along with it."

The day of my husband's funeral, my sons and my daughter came to Dallas from Houston. Perhaps it was the worst possible time to make a business decision, but it could no longer be delayed. After the funeral, we sat in my living room and discussed the recommendations I had received. My children listened in silence.

My twenty-year-old son, Richard, was a sales representative for Prudential Life Insurance Company. One of the youngest agents in Texas, he was making the incredible salary of $480 a month. (I thought that was just unbelievable—after all, he was just a kid!) If Mary Kay were to become a reality, I needed his help, but there was no way that I could afford a salary like that. I took a deep breath and offered him $250 a month to help me guide the new company. Richard accepted without hesitation. And over the horrified protests of other family members and friends, he immediately quit his job and moved to Dallas.

My elder son, Ben, was twenty-seven years old, married and the father of two. He could not pull up roots and move as quickly as his brother. But after hearing my plans to continue the company, he said, "One day I'd like to join you and Richard." Then calmly and deliberately he reached into his breast pocket and pulled out a savings passbook. The balance showed $4,500—a sum I knew represented everything he had saved since high school.

"Mother," he said, "I think you could do anything in this world that you wanted to." Then he handed me the passbook. "Here's my savings. If it will help you in any way, I want you to have it."

Eight months later—when we needed someone to handle our expanding warehouse—Ben left his job with a Houston welding company and moved his family to Dallas. He started with the company at the same pay as Richard—$250 a month. And still later, my daughter, Marylyn, joined us and became the first Mary Kay director in Houston.

On Friday, September 13, 1963, Mary Kay Cosmetics opened on schedule. With nine salespeople, my twenty-year-old son as financial administrator, and me, how did I know that I could do it? Well, I didn't! I had no crystal ball. All I knew was that I *had* to do it. As for the predictions of my attorney and accountant, I figured they didn't have any crystal balls either. Besides, they didn't understand the business the way I did. I also knew that I would never have a second chance to put my dream into action. If Mary Kay failed, I wasn't going back into an easy retirement. I'd be broke! And that meant that I'd have to work for someone else for the rest of my life. That's a very strong incentive! So no matter what anyone thought, I would not give up my dream. My children had said, "You can do it." And that was all I needed.

"You can do it!" has become an everyday motto at Mary Kay. So often a woman will join us who is in desperate need of hearing this message. She has either been out of the job market or is looking to supplement her income by building her own business. Or maybe she simply worked long and hard in another field, never having heard these words of encouragement.

If you ever come to visit Mary Kay headquarters in Dallas, you may see someone wearing a diamond pin in the shape of a bumblebee. Be assured that she is one of our top performers. Within our organization, the bumblebee has become the ultimate symbol of accomplishment. We selected it because of what the bumblebee represents for all women. You see, years ago, aerodynamic engineers studied this creature and decided that it simply *should not be able* to fly! Its wings are too weak and its body too heavy for flight. Everything seems to tell the bumblebee, "You'll never get off the ground." But I like to think that maybe—just maybe—our Divine Creator whispered, "You can do it!" So it did!

Mary Kay Ash

[EDITORS' NOTE: *Today Mary Kay Inc. is a billion-dollar company with more than 500,000 independent Beauty Consultants in twenty-seven countries. It has been recognized as "One of the 100 Best Companies to Work for in America." Mary Kay Ash has been honored with numerous awards for her efforts in helping others reach their potential. She is the only woman profiled in the book* Forbes Greatest Business Stories of All Time.]

No Mistake

In 1951, Bette Nesmith worked in a Dallas bank, where she was glad to have a secretarial job. She was twenty-seven, divorced and the mother of a nine-year-old son. She was happy to be making $300 a month, a respectable sum back then.

But she had one problem—how to correct the errors she made on her new electric typewriter. She had learned to type on a manual typewriter, and was horrified at how many more mistakes she was making on the electric. It was a nightmare trying to correct all the mistakes with an eraser. She had to figure out another way.

She had some art experience, and she knew that artists who worked in oils just painted over errors, so she concocted a fluid to paint over her typing errors, and she put it in an empty bottle of fingernail polish.

For five years, Bette kept her new technique to herself. But finally, other secretaries began to notice her little bottle, and asked for some themselves. So she made up some bottles for her friends and called it "Mistake Out."

Her friends loved it and encouraged her to start selling the product. She approached various marketing agencies and companies, including IBM, but they turned her down. However, secretaries continued to like her product, so Bette Nesmith's kitchen became her first manufacturing facility, and she started selling it on her own. She didn't quit her day job, but worked long into the nights and early mornings mixing and packaging her product.

Orders began to trickle in, and she hired a college student to help the sales effort. It wasn't easy for these two inexperienced salespeople. Dealers kept telling them that people just wouldn't paint out their mistakes. Records show that from August 1959 to April 1960, the company's total income was $1,141, and its expenses were $1,217.

But Bette didn't give up. She went to a part-time secretarial job, managing to buy groceries and save $200 to pay a chemist to develop a faster-drying formula.

The new formula helped. Bette began traveling throughout the country, selling her little white bottles wherever she could. She'd arrive in a town, get the local phone book, and call every local office supply dealer. She visited individual stores and would leave a dozen bottles. Orders mushroomed, and what had become known as Liquid Paper began to take off.

When Bette Nesmith sold her enterprise, the Liquid Paper Corporation, in 1979, the tiny white bottles were earning $3.5 million annually on sales of $38 million. The buyer was the Gillette Company, and the sale price was $47.5 million.

Jennifer Read Hawthorne and Marci Shimoff
Adapted from a story in Bits & Pieces

Police Woman

Ever since I was a little girl, I wanted to be a police officer. I was enthralled with the world of law and order. My
favorite TV show was *Police Woman*, with *The Rifleman* a
close second. Deep in my heart, I wanted to save people,
to do right; I wanted to be a hero.

I was always an overweight kid. Whenever I told my
family about my dreams of being a policewoman, they
would say, "Well, you're going to have to lose some
weight if you want to do that." I knew they were right,
and I felt ashamed of my body. But as time went on, I
didn't lose weight—I gained it.

At thirty-three, I was five foot, two inches tall and
weighed over 300 pounds. Needless to say, I hadn't
become a police officer. And of course, there was no way I
could. I was too old, too heavy—it was too ridiculous to
even consider. But deep down, it was really what I
wanted to do. Whenever I saw a cop, I felt the old thrill
and the same longing I'd had as a child.

One day I looked into the mirror, and I truly saw myself
as I was—a person with a good heart, with worthy
dreams, who had given up on herself. It was a bittersweet

moment; I felt a new tenderness, a new love for myself as well as a new honesty. I faced the woman in the mirror and asked, "How will you ever know what you can do if you don't try?"

I decided to go for it. I took the first step: the civil service exam. But test-taking has never been a strength of mine, and I failed. While it is possible to join the police force without passing the civil service exam, it is decidedly more difficult. It would have been easy to give up then, but I was determined to pursue my dream.

So, I contacted the police department in my community. I told the chief of police about my desire to join the force, and he asked to meet with me. I was very nervous about the face-to-face meeting. I kept reminding myself that what mattered was how I carried myself, my sincerity and my belief in myself. Still, I was consumed with fear and thought: *He'll take one look at me and then politely tell me, "Don't call us, we'll call you!"*

But it didn't happen that way at all. He simply accepted me, inviting me to join the police auxiliary group.

I had to get a uniform. Anticipating this task unnerved me. I would sit in my car, day after day, waiting for just the right moment to make my entrance into the police station. How would I be viewed? Would I be respected or ridiculed?

Finally, I summoned enough courage to act. Walking as tall as I could, I went inside. I wouldn't let them see my fear. With sweaty palms, I tried on uniforms, but I couldn't find any that fit me. Eventually I had to go to a tailor and have a uniform altered. How uncomfortable this was for me. While the tailor, an older man, was measuring and tucking my uniform, I could feel the temperature rising in the dressing room. I was consumed with humiliation.

I started to attend the monthly auxiliary meetings and got to know the group, all of whom were men, most of them retirees. A couple of them, like me, were working toward becoming a police officer. We met monthly, watching different movies on safety and going shooting at the range.

Soon the chief recommended me for the thirteen-week training program at the North East Regional Police Institute (NERPI). This school was demanding, both academically and physically. You had to learn criminal law, take CPR exams and learn to use handcuffs, mace spray and bayonets. I wasn't sure if I could do it—I had never stepped so far outside of my comfort zone. *How will you know what you can do—if you never try?* The thought went through my mind again, giving me just the push I needed. I would endure the fear and make myself do it.

At the school, over 90 percent of the police candidates were men under the age of twenty-five, fit and muscular. I was totally intimidated and kept to myself, trying not to imagine what those guys must have thought of me.

But the day I'd been dreading finally arrived. Working in pairs, we were going to learn how to use handcuffs. I pretended not to notice when I was the last one to be chosen as a partner. Then one person put his hands behind his back, while the partner received instructions on how to handcuff the other's wrists together. The instructor walked around, checking out each team and critiquing them in front of the entire class. Because of my size, I couldn't get my wrists together the right way so that my partner could handcuff me. The instructor was making his way over to us, and I was so anxious, the sweat was pouring down my face. I could tell my partner was uncomfortable, too, as he tried his best to coach me on ways to get my wrists closer. I prayed to somehow become invisible. But the instructor did not pass over us. Instead, he pointed out our problem to the entire class.

When it was over, I realized that my embarrassment

had been terribly uncomfortable but not fatal. The fear had been worse than the actual event. I realized it was up to me to manage the fear. The amazing thing was, I knew that I could. It was a turning point for me.

I made it through the thirteen weeks. Although test-taking and risk-taking were my constant companions, I passed all final exams, written and otherwise, with flying colors.

Now it was time to interview with a police department that didn't require the civil service test be taken or passed. Six officers conducted my interview. I began telling my story, with all the passion for the law that had always been inside of me. I held my head high and talked about making a difference in the world.

In the end, I was offered a position as police dispatcher. I wasn't exactly a policewoman, but the funny thing was, it didn't matter anymore. What mattered was that I had gone for my dreams in the face of tremendous odds. I had broken every boundary I'd held about what I could do and not do.

"How are you going to know what you can do until you try?" has become my motto. Since that time, I have let myself dream freely and pursue the dreams that really move me. I have become a motivational speaker, gone whitewater rafting, ridden motorcycles—I'm even plan-ning to go parachuting soon.

It is truly amazing what you can do—if you'll only try.

Chris Mullins

Late for School

You are never too old to set another goal or to dream a new dream.

Les Brown

All my life, I've had this recurring dream that causes me to wake up feeling strange. In it, I am a little girl again, rushing about, trying to get ready for school.

"Hurry, Gin, you'll be late for school," my mother calls to me.

"I *am* hurrying, Mom! Where's my lunch? What did I do with my books?"

Deep inside I know where the dream comes from and what it means. It is God's way of reminding me of some unfinished business in my life.

I loved everything about school, even though the school I attended in Springfield, Ohio, in the 1920s was very strict. I loved books, teachers, even tests and homework. Most of all I longed to someday march down the aisle to the strains of "Pomp and Circumstance." To me, that song was even more beautiful than "Here Comes the Bride."

But there were problems.

The Great Depression hit the hardest at large, poor families like ours. With seven children, Mom and Dad had no money for things like fine school clothes. Every morning, I cut out strips of cardboard to stuff inside my shoes to cover the holes in the soles. There was no money for musical instruments or sports uniforms or after-school treats. We sang to ourselves, played jacks or duck-on-the-rock, and munched on onions as we did homework.

These hardships I accepted. As long as I could go to school, I didn't mind too much how I looked or what I lacked.

What happened next was harder to accept. My brother Paul died of an infection after he accidentally stabbed himself in the eye with a fork. Then my father contracted tuberculosis and died. My sister, Margaret, caught the same disease, and soon she was gone, too.

The shock of these losses gave me an ulcer, and I fell behind in my schoolwork. Meanwhile, my widowed mother tried to keep going on the five dollars a week she made cleaning houses. Her face became a mask of despair.

One day I said to her, "Mom, I'm going to quit school and get a job to help out."

The look in her eyes was a mixture of grief and relief.

At fifteen, I dropped out of my beloved school and went to work in a bakery. My hope of walking down the aisle to "Pomp and Circumstance" was dead, or so I thought.

In 1940, I married Ed, a machinist, and we began our family. Then Ed decided to become a preacher, so we moved to Cincinnati, where he could attend the Cincinnati Bible Seminary. With the coming of children went the dream of schooling, forever.

Even so, I was determined that my children would have the education I had missed. I made sure the house was filled with books and magazines. I helped them with their homework and urged them to study hard. It paid off. All our six children eventually got some college training, and one of them is a college professor.

But Linda, our last child, had health problems. Juvenile arthritis in her hands and knees made it impossible for her to function in the typical classroom. Furthermore, the medications gave her cramps, stomach trouble and migraine headaches.

Teachers and principals were not always sympathetic. I lived in dread of the phone calls from school. "Mom, I'm coming home."

Now Linda was nineteen, and still she did not have her high school diploma. She was repeating my own experience.

I prayed about this problem, and when we moved to Sturgis, Michigan, in 1979, I began to see an answer. I drove to the local high school to check it out. On the bulletin board, I spotted an announcement about evening courses.

That's the answer, I said to myself. *Linda always feels better in the evening, so I'll just sign her up for night school.*

Linda was busy filling out enrollment forms when the registrar looked at me with brown, persuasive eyes and said, "Mrs. Schantz, why don't *you* come back to school?"

I laughed in his face. "Me? Ha! I'm an old woman. I'm fifty-five!"

But he persisted, and before I knew what I had done, I was enrolled for classes in English and crafts. "This is only an experiment," I warned him, but he just smiled.

To my surprise, both Linda and I thrived in evening school. I went back again the next semester, and my grades steadily improved.

It was exciting, going to school again, but it was no game. Sitting in a class full of kids was awkward, but most of them were respectful and encouraging. During the day,

I still had loads of housework to do and grandchildren to care for. Sometimes, I stayed up until two in the morning, adding columns of numbers for bookkeeping class. When the numbers didn't seem to work out, my eyes would cloud with tears and I would berate myself. *Why am I so dumb?*

But when I was down, Linda encouraged me. "Mom, you can't quit now!" And when she was down, I encouraged her. Together we would see this through.

At last, graduation was near, and the registrar called me into his office. I entered, trembling, afraid I had done something wrong.

He smiled and motioned for me to have a seat. "Mrs. Schantz," he began, "you have done very well in school."

I blushed with relief.

"As a matter of fact," he went on, "your classmates have voted unanimously for you to be class orator."

I was speechless.

He smiled again and handed me a piece of paper. "And here is a little reward for all your hard work."

I looked at the paper. It was a college scholarship for $3,000. "Thank you" was all I could think to say, and I said it over and over.

The night of graduation, I was terrified. Two hundred people were sitting out there, and public speaking was a brand-new experience for me. My mouth wrinkled as if I had been eating persimmons. My heart skipped beats, and I wanted to flee, but I couldn't! After all, my own children were sitting in that audience. I couldn't be a coward in front of them.

Then, when I heard the first strains of "Pomp and Circumstance," my fears dissolved in a flood of delight. *I am graduating! And so is Linda!*

Somehow I got through the speech. I was startled by the applause, the first I ever remember receiving in my life.

Afterwards, roses arrived from my brothers and sisters throughout the Midwest. My husband gave me silk roses, "so they will not fade."

The local media showed up with cameras and recorders and lots of questions. There were tears and hugs and congratulations. I was proud of Linda, and a little afraid that I might have unintentionally stolen some of the attention that she deserved for her victory, but she seemed as proud as anyone of our dual success.

The class of '81 is history now, and I've gone on for some college education.

But sometimes, I sit down and put on the tape of my graduation speech. I hear myself say to the audience, "Don't ever underestimate your dreams in life. Anything can happen if you believe. Not a childish, magical belief. It means hard work, but never doubt that you can do it, with God's help."

And then, I remember the recurring dream—*Hurry, Gin, you'll be late for school*—and my eyes cloud over when I think of my mother.

Yes, Mom, I was late for school, but it was all the sweeter for waiting. I only wish you and Dad could have been there to see your daughter and granddaughter in all their pomp and circumstance.

Virginia Schantz
As told to Daniel Schantz

Color My World

My husband of eleven years had left me. He hadn't just left . . . he had run away with another woman, his bookkeeper. And he hadn't just left me, he had also abandoned our four small children. My world of safe, muted colors went up in smoke with the reading of his note, and nothing remained of the woman who had been, or of my world, but gray ash.

When I took stock of myself, I saw an insecure, overweight housewife with four small children and no skills with which to support them. The two things I did have were determination and friends.

Because I was suddenly without funds, my father offered me the job of bookkeeper at the family business— at the farm implement dealership he co-owned with my husband. I was to replace the woman who had run off with my husband. Though determined to keep my kids afloat, it seemed a cruel joke that I had to go in every day, sit at *her* desk, answer *her* phone, and try to do *her* bookkeeping job.

The farmers who came in winced at the sight of me. Everyone was aware of the story, aware of my pain. The humiliation made me sick to my stomach every day. I was so insecure that going to the mailbox or the grocery store took all my energy.

Where only a week before, my quiet days had been spent looking after the children, cooking, cleaning and knitting, I was suddenly thrown out into the working world, unprepared.

After a few weeks, I decided that if I had to work as a bookkeeper, I would learn how to do the job correctly. I enrolled in a night class in accounting. I hated it. Numbers had never been my thing, and being in class with all those bright young people unnerved me. But I was determined to make a life for my children at any cost.

After I successfully passed that first course, my father offered to buy out my half of the business so I could go to school full-time. This meant I would have an income while attending classes. By the time the payments ended, I could have my degree and, hopefully, a high-paying job.

When I timidly mentioned this offer to my friend Robbie, she enthusiastically said she'd help in any way she could. And she did! Within days, we were maneuvering the parking lots of the nearby community college and marching toward the registrar's office, where I signed up for accounting classes. I was going to be an accountant—me, who had always hated numbers!

Robbie said that we needed to celebrate this first step toward a new life, so we stopped at a restaurant for lunch. There, we met another old friend, JoAnn, who had been a commercial artist. She was now painting her own water-colors and taught art classes—in fact, her classes had been one of my few indulgences between my first two babies. Like everyone else in town, JoAnn had heard about my plight and asked how I was doing. At least there was something new to tell.

"She's going back to school!" Robbie grinned.

"Oh!" my former teacher exclaimed. "You're finally going to get into graphic design!"

"No," I stammered. "Actually, I've just signed up for accounting courses."

"Oh?" She was clearly confused.

I was stunned. It had never occurred to me to go to school for something I *wanted* to do. Since my husband's disappearance, I had plodded along, doing whatever was necessary, going through the motions of my life.

As we drove home, I thought about the possibility of changing my major. I reopened the catalog in my lap to the section describing graphic design. The course names danced before me as I read them to Robbie: "Illustration! Art history! Oil painting! Can this be a real career?" I gasped in awe.

"Thank God!" Robbie was now laughing. "I was beginning to think that this was all just wasted effort. I haven't seen you excited about anything in months!"

That evening, I gathered my courage and called JoAnn at her home. "Do you think I could support my children with graphic design?" I asked.

"I did it. And you are good . . . very good! I really believe that you could do it, too," she answered, and it sounded as if there was even relief in her voice.

The next day, I marched back to college—on my own. When I said I was changing my major, the course counselor looked at me as if I'd lost my mind.

It turned out to be one of the best choices I've ever made.

And you know what? I am actually thankful for my first marriage and for having to live through such traumatic times. If not for that marriage, I would not have my wonderful children. If I had not had to struggle, I might still be thinking of myself as an unhappy, overweight housewife, afraid to leave the house.

Instead, I went on to earn the prestigious title of creative director with a large company, and the paycheck to go with it. My studio wall is lined with awards, which I consider medals of honor in my long-fought battle. I was able to put all my children through college; they are now grown with families and careers of their own. We are closer and stronger for having shared, and overcome, that time of pain.

But most of all, the colors of my life are not muted, nor did they remain gray ash forever. The spectrum is full and the colors are vibrant! I might never have known that this rainbow of strength and love was inside me all along. Every day, I thank God for the small kernel of determination—and the support of my friends—who helped find and free the rainbow during that stormiest of times.

Sharon M. Chamberlain

He Taught Me to Fly

*Everyone should carefully observe which way
his heart draws him, and then choose that way
with all his strength.*

Hasidic Saying

My dad grew up not far from the Cabrini Green housing project in Chicago. The projects were built long after Dad moved out, but the tough, teeming neighborhood of his youth is not so very different from the neighborhood of today. It's still a place for people trying to find a way out of poverty and danger. To finally see that apartment house was to finally know the deepest part of my father. It was to finally understand why we spent so much time at odds.

Dad and I were always passionate about our feelings—we're Italian, after all—and when I reached my teen years, our arguments really heated up. I can't remember a meal from those years that we didn't argue through. Politics, feminism, the war in Vietnam. Our biggest fight, however, was an ongoing one. It was about my chosen profession.

"People like us aren't writers!" Dad would shout.

"Maybe people like *you* aren't writers," I would shoot back, "but people like *me* are!"

What I said was truer than I knew.

I grew up in a nice house with a lawn, a dog and lots of room to stretch out in. My only responsibilities were to get good grades and stay out of major trouble. Dad spent his youth squeezed into a tenement, taking care of a widowed mother who spoke no English, helping to parent two younger siblings—and earning enough money in whatever way he could to keep the family going.

Dad's dream was to move up and out of the old neighborhood, and after he married, he did. He drew a curtain over his past, never speaking of his growing-up days. Not to anyone. Ever. It was a point of pride with him that he allowed no one to know what he had suffered through. But by not knowing Dad's past, I could never really know him, or what drove him to want so much security for me.

As I persisted in my career, despite all the rejections, Mom told me Dad read and re-read everything I got published, although he never mentioned my work to me. Instead, he continually tried to steer me into a career he considered far safer—nursing or teaching or secretarial.

But in the last week of his life, as I sat by his bed, Dad opened up. It was as if he suddenly realized that soon it would be too late to let anyone know the truth. That's when he had me dig out a box of pictures he'd buried deep in the garage; that's when I finally saw what he and his brother and sister had looked like as children, and where they had lived. It was when I came face to face not only with Dad's old home, but with my father himself.

In those last days, Dad talked about everything. How it felt to carry buckets of coal up four flights of stairs and share one bathroom with five other families. He told me that he was always worried that his brother and sister wouldn't have enough to eat or that they wouldn't have enough warm clothes for winter, or that someone in the family would get sick and there wouldn't be enough money for medicine or doctors. He told me about the Saturdays he spent on a country club golf course, how wonderful the grass looked to him, and how he tried to get the men to use him as a caddie. After eighteen holes, if he was lucky, they'd toss him a quarter.

Dad told me how he'd wanted to protect me from poverty and want, so I'd never have to go through what he had. He told me how important it was to him that I have something to fall back on. And I told Dad that what I'd fallen back on all these years was him. I told him my hopes and dreams had been built on his strong shoulders. I told him the roots he'd given me ran deep, and when he apologized for trying to clip my wings, I told him that he was the one who'd given me the chance to fly. Dad smiled at that and tried to nod, but I wasn't sure if he'd really understood what I'd meant.

But on the afternoon of the last day of his life, as Mom and I sat holding his hands, he beckoned the two hospice volunteers close. "You know my daughter," he whispered with great effort. "Well, I just want you to know—she's a writer."

It was the proudest moment of my life.

Cynthia Mercati

4

ON MARRIAGE

How do I love thee? Let me count the ways.
I love thee to the depth and breadth and
height my soul can reach . . .

Elizabeth Barrett Browning

The Real Thing

If I know what love is, it is because of you.

Herman Hesse

Cecile and I have been friends since college, for more than thirty years. Although we have never lived closer than 100 miles to each other, since we first met, our friendship has remained constant. We have seen each other through marriage, birth, divorce, the death of loved ones—all those times when you really need a friend.

In celebration of our friendship and our fiftieth birthday, Cecile and I took our first road trip together. We drove from my home in Texas to California and back. What a wonderful time we had!

The first day of our trip ended in Santa Fe, New Mexico. After the long drive, we were quite tired, so we decided to go to the restaurant near the hotel for dinner. We were seated in a rather quiet part of the dining room with only a few other patrons. We ordered our food and settled back to recount our day. As we talked, I glanced at the other people in the room. I noticed an attractive elderly couple sitting a short distance away from us. The gentleman was rather tall and athletic looking, with silver hair and a tanned complexion. The lady seated beside him was petite, well-dressed and lovely. What caught my immediate attention was the look of adoration on the woman's face. She sat, chin resting gently on her hands, and stared into the face of the man as he talked. She reminded me of a teenager in love!

I called Cecile's attention to the couple. As we watched, he reached over to place a gentle kiss on her cheek. She smiled.

"Now that's what I call real love!" I said with a sigh. "I imagine they've been married for a long time. They look so in love!"

"Or maybe," remarked Cecile, "they haven't been together long. It could be they've just fallen in love."

"Well, whatever the case, it's obvious they care a great deal for each other. They are in love."

Cecile and I watched surreptitiously and unashamedly eavesdropped on their conversation. He was explaining to her about a new business investment he was considering and asking her opinion. She smiled and agreed with whatever he said. When the waitress came to take their order, he ordered for her, reminding her that the veal was her favorite. He caressed her hand as he talked, and she listened raptly to his every word. We were enthralled by the poignant scene we were witnessing.

Then the scene changed. A perplexed look came over the finely wrinkled but beautiful face. She looked at the man and said in a sweet voice, "Do I know you? What is this place? Where are we?"

"Now, sweetheart, you know me. I'm Ralph, your husband. And we're in Santa Fe. We are going to see our son in Missouri tomorrow. Don't you remember?"

"Oh, I'm not sure. I seem to have forgotten," she said quietly.

"That's okay, sweetheart. You'll be all right. Just eat your dinner, and we'll go and get some rest." He reached over and caressed her cheek. "You sure do look pretty tonight."

Tears coursed down our cheeks as Cecile and I looked at each other. "We were right," she said quietly. "It is the real thing. That is love."

Frankie Germany

The Locket

As a seminar leader, I hear a lot of stories about people's lives and experiences. One day at the end of a seminar, a woman came up to me and told me about an event that changed her life—and in the telling, touched mine.

"I used to think I was just a nurse," she began, "until one day a couple of years ago.

"It was noontime and I was feeding 'the feeders,' the elderly who cannot feed themselves. Messy work, keeping track of each one and making sure they keep the food in their mouths. I looked up as an elderly gentleman passed by the dining room doorway. He was on his way down the hall for a daily visit with his wife.

"Our eyes met over the distance, and I knew right then in my heart that I should be with them both that noon hour. My coworker covered for me, and I followed him down the corridor.

"When I entered the room, she was lying in bed, looking up at the ceiling with her arms across her chest. He was sitting in the chair at the end of the bed with his arms crossed, looking at the floor.

"I walked over to her and said, 'Susan, is there anything you want to share today? If so, I came down to listen.' She tried to speak but her lips were dry and nothing came out. I bent over closer and asked again.

"'Susan, if you cannot say it with words, can you show me with your hands?'

"She carefully lifted her hands off her chest and held them up before her eyes. They were old hands, with leathery skin and swollen knuckles, worn from years of caring, working and living. She then grasped the collar of her nightgown and began to pull.

"I unbuttoned the top buttons. She reached in and pulled out a long gold chain connected to a small gold locket. She held it up, and tears came to her eyes.

"Her husband got up from the end of the bed and came over. Sitting beside her, he took his hands and tenderly placed them around hers. 'There is a story about this locket,' he explained, and he began to tell it to me.

"'One day many months ago, we awoke early and I told Susan I could no longer care for her by myself. I could not carry her to the bathroom, keep the house clean, plus cook all the meals. My body could no longer do this. I, too, had aged.

"'We talked long and hard that morning. She told me to go to coffee club and ask where a good place might be. I didn't return until lunch time. We chose here from the advice of others.

"'On the first day, after all the forms, the weighing and the tests, the nurse told us that her fingers were so swollen that they would need to cut off her wedding rings.

"'After everyone left the room, we sat together and she asked me, "What do we do with a broken ring and a whole ring?" For I had chosen to take off my ring that day, too.

"'Both of these rings were old, more oval than round.

Thin in some places and strong in other parts. We made a difficult decision. That was the hardest night in my entire life. It was the first time we had slept apart in forty-three years.

"'The next morning I took the two rings to the jewelers and had them melted. Half of that locket is my ring, and the other half is hers. The clasp is made from the engagement ring that I gave her when I proposed to her, down by the pond at the back of the farm on a warm summer's evening. She told me it was about time and answered yes.

"'On the inside it says *I love you Susan* and on the other side it says *I love you Joseph*. We made this locket because we were afraid that one day we might not be able to say these words to each other.'

"He picked her up and held her gently in his arms. I knew that I was the channel, and they had the message. I slipped out the door and went back to feeding the feeders with more kindness in my heart.

"After lunch and the paperwork, I walked back down to their room. He was rocking her in his arms and singing the last verse of 'Amazing Grace.' I waited while he laid her down, crossed her arms and closed her eyes.

"He turned to me at the door and said, 'Thank you. She passed away just a little bit ago. Thank you very much.'

"I used to say I was 'just a nurse' or 'just a mom,' but I don't anymore. No one is just an anything. Each of us has gifts and talents. We need not limit ourselves by such small definitions. I know what I can do when I listen to my heart and live from there."

As she finished her story, we hugged and she left. I stood in the doorway with thankfulness.

Geery Howe

The Dowry

In the faraway world of the South Pacific, there is an island named Nurabandi and, nearby, another one called Kiniwata.

The natives of these islands are all said to be very wonderful, to be fine and proud, but they still hold to the ageless custom of offering a dowry to a girl's family when a young man asks for her hand in marriage.

Johnny Lingo lived on the island of Nurabandi. He was handsome and rich and perhaps the smartest businessman on the entire island. Everyone knew that Johnny, a young bachelor, could have his pick of just about any of the single girls in the region.

But Johnny only had eyes for Sarita, who lived on Kiniwata, and some people had a hard time figuring that out.

Sarita, you see, was a rather plain, homely looking girl. When she walked, her shoulders slumped and her head ducked down just so.

Nonetheless, Johnny was deeply in love with Sarita and made arrangements to meet Sarita's father, a man named Sam Karoo, to ask for her hand in marriage and to discuss a proper dowry.

Now, the dowry was always paid in live cows because the animals were at such a premium on the small islands of the Pacific rim. History showed that some of the most beautiful South Pacific girls went for a dowry of four cows or, in a really rare instance, five.

Further, Johnny Lingo was the shrewdest trader on the island of Nurabandi and Sarita's daddy, bless his heart, was the worst of anyone on the island of Kiniwata.

Knowing this, a worried Sam Karoo sat down with his family the night before the now-famous meeting and nervously plotted his strategy: He'd ask Johnny for three cows, but hold out for two until they were sure Johnny would give one.

The next day, at the very start of the meeting, Johnny Lingo looked Sam Karoo right in the eye and said evenly, "I would like to offer you eight cows as I ask your daughter, Sarita, to marry me."

Well, Sam stammered that would be just fine. Soon there was a dandy wedding, but nobody on any of the islands could figure out why on earth Johnny gave eight cows for Sarita.

Six months later, an American visitor, a gifted writer named Pat McGerr, met with Johnny Lingo at his beautiful home on Nurabandi and asked about the eight cows.

The writer had already been to the island of Kiniwata and had heard the villagers there still giggling over the fact that stupid ol' Sam had duped the wise Johnny out of eight cows for the homely and plain Sarita.

Yet in Nurabandi, no one dared laugh at Johnny Lingo because he was held in such high esteem. When the writer finally met Johnny, the new husband's eyes twinkled as he gently questioned the writer.

"I hear they speak of me on that island. My wife is from there."

"Yes, I know," said the writer.

"So, tell me, what do they say?" asked Johnny.

The writer, struggling to be diplomatic, replied, "Well, that you were married to Sarita at festival time."

Johnny pressed on and on until the writer finally told him candidly, "They say you gave eight cows for your wife, and they wonder why you did that."

Right then, the most beautiful woman the writer had ever seen came into the room to put flowers on the table.

She was tall. And her shoulders were square. And her chin was straight. And, when her eyes caught Johnny's, there was an undeniable spark.

"This is my wife, Sarita," the now-amused Johnny said, and as Sarita excused herself, the writer was mystified.

And then Johnny began to explain.

"Do you ever think what it must mean to a woman to know her husband settled on the lowest price for which she could be bought?

"And then later, when the women talk among themselves, they boast what their husbands paid for them. One says four cows, another says three. But how does the woman feel who is bought for only one?" said Johnny.

"I wasn't going to let that happen to my Sarita. I wanted Sarita to be happy, yes, but it was more than that. You say she is different than you were told. That is true, but many things change a woman.

"Things happen inside and things happen outside, but what's most important is what she thinks about herself. In Kiniwata, Sarita believed she was worth nothing, but now she knows she is worth more than any woman on any of the islands."

Johnny Lingo paused just so and then added, "I wanted to marry Sarita from the beginning. I loved her and no other woman. But I also wanted to have an eight-cow wife, and, so you see, my dream came true."

Roy Exum

Going the Right Way

In 1939, in a small town in Oklahoma, a young couple had been married a few short and disappointing months. He never dreamed there were so many ways to ruin fried chicken. She couldn't imagine why she ever thought his jokes were funny. Neither one said aloud what they were both thinking—the marriage was a big mistake.

One hot afternoon, they got into a terrible argument about whether they could afford to paint the living room. Tempers flared, voices were raised, and somehow one of the wedding gift plates crashed to the floor. She burst into tears, called him heartless and a cheapskate. He shouted that he'd rather be a cheapskate than a nag, then grabbed the car keys on his way out. His parting words, punctuated by the slam of the screen door, were, "That's it! I'm leaving you!"

But before he could coax their rickety car into gear, the passenger door flew open and his bride landed on the seat beside him. She stared straight ahead, her face tear-streaked but determined.

"And just where do you think *you're* going?" he asked in amazement.

She hesitated only a moment before replying, just long enough to be sure of the answer that would decide the direction of their lives for the next forty-three years.

"If you're leaving me," my mother said, "I'm going with you."

Lynne Kinghorn

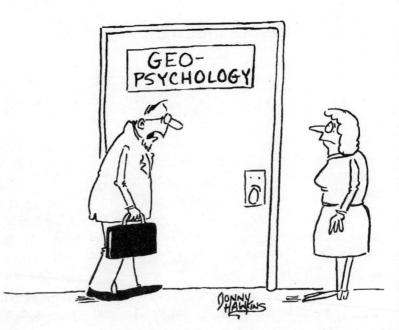

"I specialize in rocky relationships."

Reprinted by permission of Jonny Hawkins.

I'll Never Understand My Wife

In every union there is a mystery.

Henri F. Amiel

I'll never understand my wife.

The day she moved in with me, she started opening and closing my kitchen cabinets, gasping, "You don't have any shelf paper! We're going to have to get some shelf paper in here before I move my dishes in."

"But why?" I asked innocently.

"To keep the dishes clean," she answered matter-of-factly. I didn't understand how the dust would magically migrate off the dishes if they had sticky blue paper under them, but I knew when to be quiet.

Then came the day when I left the toilet seat up.

"We never left the toilet seat up in my family," she scolded. "It's impolite."

"It wasn't impolite in my family," I said sheepishly.

"You're family didn't have cats."

In addition to these lessons, I also learned how I was supposed to squeeze the toothpaste tube, which towel to use after a shower and where the spoons are supposed to go when I set the table. I had no idea I was so uneducated.

Nope, I'll never understand my wife.

She alphabetizes her spices, washes dishes before sending them through the dishwasher, and sorts laundry into different piles before throwing it into the washing machine. Can you imagine?

She wears pajamas to bed. I didn't think anyone in North America still wore pajamas to bed. She has a coat that makes her look like Sherlock Holmes. "I could get you a new coat," I offered.

"No. This one was my grandmother's," she said, decisively ending the conversation.

Then, after we had kids, she acted even stranger. Wearing those pajamas all day long, eating breakfast at 1:00 P.M., carrying around a diaper bag the size of a minivan, talking in one syllable paragraphs.

She carried our baby everywhere—on her back, on her front, in her arms, over her shoulder. She never set her down, even when other young mothers shook their heads as they set down the car seat with their baby in it, or peered down into their playpens. What an oddity she was, clutching that child.

My wife also chose to nurse her even when her friends told her not to bother. She picked up the baby whenever she cried, even though people told her it was healthy to let her wail.

"It's good for her lungs to cry," they would say.

"It's better for her heart to smile," she'd answer.

One day a friend of mine snickered at the bumper sticker my wife had put on the back of our car: "Being a Stay-at-Home Mom Is a Work of Heart."

"My wife must have put that on there," I said.

"My wife works," he boasted.

"So does mine," I said, smiling.

Once, I was filling out one of those warranty registration cards and I checked "homemaker" for my wife's occupation. Big mistake. She glanced over it and quickly corrected me. "I am not a homemaker. I am not a housewife. I am a mother."

"But there's no category for that," I stammered.

"Add one," she said.

I did.

And then one day, a few years later, she lay in bed smiling when I got up to go to work.

"What's wrong?" I asked.

"Nothing. Everything is wonderful. I didn't have to get up at all last night to calm the kids. And they didn't crawl in bed with us."

"Oh," I said, still not understanding.

"It was the first time I've slept through the night in four years." It was? Four years? That's a long time. I hadn't even noticed. Why hadn't she ever complained? I would have.

One day, in one thoughtless moment, I said something that sent her fleeing to the bedroom in tears. I went in to apologize. She knew I meant it because by then I was crying, too.

"I forgive you," she said. And you know what? She did. She never brought it up again. Not even when she got angry and could have hauled out the heavy artillery. She forgave, and she forgot.

Nope, I'll never understand my wife. And you know what? Our daughter is acting more and more like her mother every day.

If she turns out to be anything like her mom, someday there's going be one more lucky guy in this world, thankful for the shelf paper in his cupboard.

Steven James

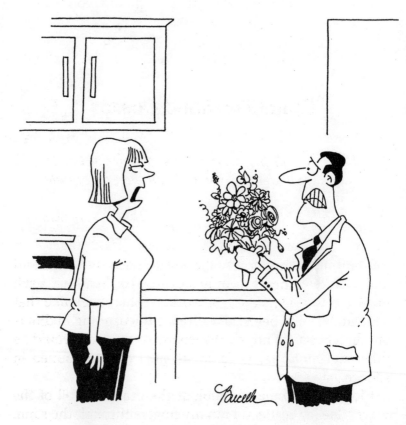

"No, I'm not happy you bought me flowers for
absolutely no reason. It's our anniversary."

Crumbling Sand Castles

Love doesn't just sit there like a stone; it has to be made, like bread, remade all the time, made new.

Ursula K. Le Guin

One mild summer day beside the sea, my husband and I were lying on our beach towels, reading, each locked in our own separate worlds. It had been like that a lot lately. We'd been busy, preoccupied, going in different directions. I'd hoped the leisure of vacation would be different, but so far we'd spent most of it marooned in silence.

I looked up from my book at the ceaseless roll of the waves, feeling restless. I ran my fingers through the sand. "Want to make a sand castle?" I asked my husband.

He didn't really, but he humored me. Once we got started, though, he became surprisingly absorbed in the project. We both did. In fact, after a while we were working over that heap of beach sand as if it was about to be photographed for *Sand Castle Digest*. Sandy made bridges across the moat, while I crowned the top of the castle with spires. We made balconies and arched windows lined with tiny angel-wing shells. It looked like Camelot.

Neither of us noticed when the tide changed. We never saw the waves slipping up until the first swish of water gnawed a little piece of our castle away. Indignant, we shored it up with sand and patted it down. But as the waves returned with monotonous regularity, our hands grew still and our eyes drifted off toward the horizon. Sandy got on his beach towel. I got on mine. We went back to our silence.

The next time I looked around, the sand castle we'd labored over was awash in the shifting tide. The bridges were washing away and the spires were starting to lean.

I gave it a soulful look, an inexplicable sadness coming over me. And suddenly in the midst of that ordinary summer, I had a moment of pure, unbidden revelation. *There sits my marriage,* I thought.

I looked at my husband. The soundlessness between us seemed to reach clear to the sky. It was the hollow silence of a mid-life marriage, a marriage in which the ceaseless noise of everyday living threatens to drown out the music of intimacy.

Dear God, when had the tide shifted? When had mortgages and laundry and orthodontist appointments become more important than those unspeakably long looks we used to exchange! How long since we'd shared our hidden pain or stumbled together upon a joy that was round with wonder and laughter? How had it happened that two people who loved each other could allow such distance to creep in!

I thought of the attentiveness we'd lavished upon our relationship in the beginning, and how, eventually, the endless demands and routines of running a household, raising two children, and juggling two careers had stilled our hands and averted our eyes.

That night, after the children were asleep, my husband found me standing in the shadows on the porch, staring at the night. "You've hardly said two words all evening."

"Sorry," I muttered. "I've just got something on my mind."

"You want to tell me what it is?" he asked.

I turned around and looked at him. I took a deep breath. "I'm thinking of us," I said. "I'm thinking that our relationship is being drowned out by the demands of day-to-day living. We've taken our marriage for granted."

"What are you talking about? We have a very committed marriage." He was indignant.

"Of course we have a committed marriage," I told him. "But sometimes it seems commitment is all we've got. Sometimes we are two strangers existing under one roof, each going separate ways."

He didn't say a word. *Now I've done it,* I thought. *I've rocked the boat to the point of tipping over. I've told my husband our marriage is bordering on empty commitment. Good grief!* We stared at each other. It was as if we were stuck inside some big, dark bubble of pain that wouldn't pop. Tears welled up in my eyes and started down my face. To my amazement, tears slid down his face, too.

And suddenly, in what is surely the most endearing moment of my marriage, Sandy took his finger and traced the path of tears on my cheeks, then touched his own wet face, blending our tears together.

Strange how such things can begin to re-create the mystery of relatedness between two people. Sandy and I walked down the porch steps onto the beach under the blazing stars. Slowly we started to talk. We talked a long time. About the small agonies of being married, about the struggle of it all. We talked about the gnawed and fraying places in our marriage and how they'd happened. We spoke aching words about the unmet needs between us.

We were whirling in the darkness that had settled in our relationship. And yes, it was uncomfortable and scary, like bobbing around in the ocean without a boat. But trading chaos and braving pain is often the only way to come upon a new shoreline. For God is in dark water, too.

Finally, with the hour late and a sense of deepening and newness growing between us, I said rather dreamily, "It might be nice someday to say our wedding vows to each other again."

"What's wrong with right now?" my husband asked. I swallowed. Was there no end to the surprises this man would spring on me tonight!

"B-But what would we say! I mean, I can't remember the vows exactly."

"Why don't we simply say what's in our hearts?"

So out there beneath the light of the stars, with the crash of waves filling the night, we took each other's hand and tried to put words to the music we had begun to recapture between us.

"I promise to listen to you," he said. "To make time for genuine sharing ... "

"And I promise to be honest, to work at creating more togetherness between us," I began.

I don't remember all the words; mostly I remember the feelings behind them, the way my voice quivered and his hand tightened over mine. Mostly I thought that what we were doing was rebuilding the castle, restoring the bridges, raising the spires.

The next morning we left the children stationed in front of the television with their breakfast cereal and went walking along the ocean edge. The sun poured a golden dial of light across the water that seemed to point us on and on. We talked as we went, a little awed by the events of the night before—knowing in the harsh light of day that saying words is one thing, but living them is another.

We couldn't leave our newly spoken vows back there dripping in the moonlight. We had to take them home to the frantic schedules and the broken dryer and the Dorito crumbs under my son's bed.

Miles down the beach we waded knee-high into the surf and stood soaking up the turquoise sky and jade water. We were about to turn back to the condo when it happened. A huge, bottle-nosed dolphin came splashing out of the water a mere twenty yards away, startling us so badly we fell backward into the surf.

Sitting in the water fully clothed . . . a dolphin diving and surfacing before us in a spinning silver dance, was such an unexpected and exhilarating wonder, the two of us laughed until our insides hurt. I cannot remember a joy ever so plump and full.

At last we picked our delirious selves up and walked in our soggy shorts back up the beach, where a few crumbling sand castles dotted the shore. I took note of each one of them.

And I began to hear a voice deep inside me whispering: "When tomorrow comes and life beats upon your castle walls, remember the power of honest pain and blended tears. Remember the healing of laughter deeply shared. Remember what's important. Hold onto it always."

Sue Monk Kidd

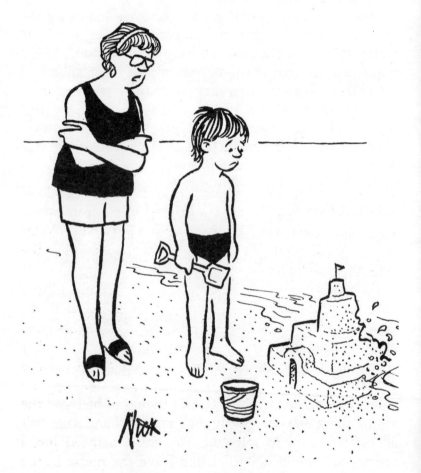

"Honey, you forgot the first rule
of real estate—location."

Reprinted by permission of Nick Hobart.

The Last "I Love You"

Carol's husband was killed in an accident last year. Jim, only fifty-two years old, was driving home from work. The other driver was a teenager with a very high blood-alcohol level. Jim died instantly. The teenager was in the emergency room for less than two hours.

There were other ironic twists: It was Carol's fiftieth birthday, and Jim had two plane tickets to Hawaii in his pocket. He was going to surprise her. Instead, he was killed by a drunk driver.

"How have you survived this?" I finally asked Carol, a year later.

Her eyes welled up with tears. I thought I had said the wrong thing, but she gently took my hand and said, "It's all right; I want to tell you. The day I married Jim, I promised I would never let him leave the house in the morning without telling him I loved him. He made the same promise. It got to be a joke between us, and as babies came along, it got to be a hard promise to keep. I remember running down the driveway, saying 'I love you' through clenched teeth when I was mad, or driving to the office to put a note in his car. It was a funny challenge.

"We made a lot of memories trying to say 'I love you' before noon every day of our married life.

"The morning Jim died, he left a birthday card in the kitchen and slipped out to the car. I heard the engine starting. *Oh, no, you don't, buster,* I thought. I raced out and banged on the car window until he rolled it down.

"'Here on my fiftieth birthday, Mr. James E. Garret, I, Carol Garret, want to go on record as saying I love you!'

"That's how I've survived. Knowing that the last words I said to Jim were *'I love you.'* "

Debbi Smoot

Loving Donna

It has been said that love is not something you find; it's something you do. Loving Donna is the easiest thing I've ever done in my life.

We've been married to each other for twenty-one years, and we're still newlyweds, if you consider that marriage is supposed to be forever.

A year ago, when the phone rang and I answered it, the voice said, "This is Doctor Freeman. Your wife has breast cancer." He spoke matter-of-factly, not mincing any words, although I could tell from his tone that he was not in a matter-of-fact frame of mind. He is a warm, caring and kindly physician, and this was not an easy phone call to make. He talked to Donna for a few minutes, and when she hung up the phone, the color drained from her face, and we held each other and cried for about five minutes.

She sighed and said, "That's enough of that."

I looked at her. "Okay," I said. "We have cancer. We'll handle it."

In the twelve months since then, Donna has had chemotherapy, a mastectomy, a bone-marrow transplant and radiation. She lost her hair, she lost a breast, she lost her privacy, and she lost the comfort associated with the assumption that tomorrow always comes. Suddenly, all her tomorrows were put on hold, and doled out, piecemeal, until the supply could be reestablished.

But she never lost her dignity or her faith. She never gave up, and she never gave in.

We put a small sign on the wall beside her bed. It said: "Sometimes the Lord calms the storm. Sometimes he lets the storm rage and calms his child." The words of the small sign became our anthem.

The day she returned home after her mastectomy, she looked at herself in the mirror, carefully. Then she shrugged, said, "So that's what I look like," put on her pajamas and got into bed. She looked at herself and saw hope; I saw courage.

She was in the hospital for Easter, Mother's Day and a high school graduation. She missed a lot of other people's lives during an interminable list of medical procedures.

But she gained a lot, too.

She attended the wedding of one of our sons in a motorized wheelchair, wearing a wig and a padded bra, and, next to the bride, she was undoubtedly the most radiant woman there.

And she found out how much her extended family and her neighbors loved her, and how much she meant in the lives of all of us. We received notes and letters and phone calls and mysterious packages of homemade bread and cookies left on our doorstep. Donna said she didn't realize how many people cared about her.

One night, at the lowest point of her physical ordeal, I was in my usual chair in the quiet of her hospital room. She had finished four days of around-the-clock high-dose chemotherapy. Her immune system had been destroyed. Her head was shiny-bald, her eyes glassy, her body thirty pounds lighter and wracked with waves of nausea. She woke up, and I reached over to touch her hand. I held it, gently, because her skin and veins and every part of her body were as fragile as the petals of a gardenia. If the bone marrow transplant didn't engraft, this was the beginning of the end. If the transplant worked, this was the bottom, and she could start climbing the steep road to recovery.

"Hi," I said. "I love you."

She laughed. "Yeah, sure you do. I'll bet you say that to all your girlfriends."

"Of course I do. Because you're all my girlfriends."

She smiled, the sedatives took over again, and she went back to sleep. Mercifully, she spent most of that week in a drug-induced mental twilight.

Ten days later, her bone marrow had engrafted, and her body was beginning to restore itself. A wonderful volunteer named Nancy came by Donna's room to teach her how to watercolor as part of her recovery therapy. I was in the room, and the lady handed me a brush and paper and paints with the simple command, "Paint something."

I have a great eye for beauty. I know it when I see it. But since elementary school, when I was young and innocent enough to believe that everything I painted was a work of art, I have learned that my hand-eye coordination is limited to the use of a computer keyboard and the TV remote control. I don't draw, and I don't paint.

So I dabbed some colors on the page, and I painted a bouquet of flowers that I pretended was something in the style that Picasso might have done and called "cubist" or Grandma Moses might have done and called "primitive." I was encouraged when Donna and Nancy both recognized them as daffodils, and that they could see seven of them, which is what I had intended.

I had remembered some lyrics from an old ballad that I'd heard more than forty years ago, so I wrote them on the bottom of the picture. I said:

I haven't any mansion;
I haven't any land.
Not one paper dollar to crinkle in my hand.
But I can show you mornings on a thousand hills,
And kiss you, and give you
Seven daffodils.

She put my picture on the wall in her room, and it was like seeing my childhood dreams stuck to the refrigerator door once again. Only this time, it was about life and death and love and hope.

She's home now, and life goes on for us. Every day we laugh a little and sometimes we cry a little. And we love a lot.

I love her for all the best reasons that a man loves a woman. In the end, I love her because she makes more of my world and my life than I can make of them by myself.

She loves me for all the simple reasons that a woman loves a man. For quiet nights and sunny days. For shared laughter and common tears. For twenty-one years of dishes and diapers and going to work and coming home and seeing her own future when she looks into my eyes.

And for a picture of seven daffodils.

Ron C. Eggertsen

History and Chemistry

I heard some women talking in the beauty shop the other day, commiserating with one another because the romance, the spark, the zip had gone out of their marriages. There was no excitement anymore, they said, no spark.

"That's life," one said. "It's inevitable. Time passes. Things change."

"I'd like to have that chemistry back," another said, sighing. "I envy young lovers. Violins and fireworks."

I thought back to those early days of my own special romance, when I floated, rather than walked. I never got hungry and frequently forgot to eat. My hair was shiny, my skin was clear and I was considerate, warm-hearted and unfailingly good-humored. When my true love and I were apart, I spent every miserable moment thinking about him. I was wretched until we were together again, sometimes as long as two or three hours. Life was one glorious rush after another—when the phone would ring, or I'd hear him at the door, or when our hands would accidentally touch.

Now, this is the same man who today, remembers our

wedding anniversary no more often than once every five years, who rarely closes a cupboard door or a drawer after he has opened one, and who resists replenishing his wardrobe until I have to secretly get rid of his more disreputable things to maintain family dignity.

I wouldn't say he's predictable, but he asks, "What did you make for lunch?" six days out of seven, after we agreed, upon his retirement, it was every person for himself at lunch time. Most recently he repeatedly asked, "What do you want for your birthday?" so often that finally, worn down, I named something. He gave me something else.

He enjoys TV or movies only if they have car chases, explosions or shootings every seven minutes, and then only at ear-shattering volume. He considers it his right, by virtue of being born male, to control the TV channel selector, and is hormonally incapable of speaking softly or closing the front door without causing the whole house to shudder.

However . . . this is also the man who, when I decide to go on a diet, says, "Why? You look good to me." Who gets out of bed on a chilly night to put an extra blanket on the bed because he knows I'm cold. Who gave me a stunning necklace for my above-mentioned birthday after I asked for foul-weather boating gear, telling me I should "just go ahead and get that other stuff" myself.

He's a man with more integrity in his little finger than anyone I've ever known to have in their entire body, and who recently bragged to my in-laws that I supported him in the early, lean years of his career—thirty-four years after the fact. He's a man who, in spite of his own personal frugality left over from his poverty-stricken era, loans large sums of money to our adult children at the drop of a hat, with no time limits and no interest payments. He can always be counted on to be there in a crisis, to be calm, rational, strong, fair and loving. Over the years, he has held me in his arms when my mother died, has held my head when I threw up, my hand when I labored to give birth to our children, and my heart from the first time I saw him.

I remembered the women in the beauty shop the other day as I sat in the car waiting for him to return from an errand across the street. I caught a glimpse of a slender, good-looking, vigorous man on the sidewalk. His head was lowered, hands in his pockets as he walked along, whistling. Very appealing. He raised his head and grinned. Zing!

The father of my children. The other name on my checking account. The man I fell in love with.

History and chemistry. It just doesn't get any better.

E. Lynne Wright

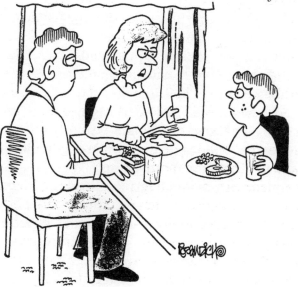

"Don't interrupt your father when he's listening to me."

True Intimacy

*Love cures people—both the ones who give it
and the ones who receive it.*

Karl Menninger

After two twelve-hour surgeries in seven days to rebuild
my degenerating spine, all I remember is pain. The maximum pain medications barely dented my agony and, in my
daze, I thought surely the entire ordeal would kill me.

The day came when I had no words, no identity, no reason left, so I screamed. I remember none of it, but I am
sure it was one of those times when I fought everything I
could fight, and screaming rolled out like a war cry. And I
thrashed, threatening to pull tubes and needles out of
arms, neck and legs.

My husband, because he loved me and suffered with
me, held my hand, paced, felt powerless and pled with
God to remove my agony and give it to him. The nurse,
starched and efficient, bent over me and said to take some
deep breaths and stop fighting. As she explained crisply,
"You will hurt yourself and undo the surgery done to help
you. So stop, or we'll have to stop you."

It was like speaking to me in another language that I neither understood nor cared to learn. Somewhere inside the fire raging in my body, her words only made me fight harder.

Finally, to my husband, she said, "Listen, I know this must be very hard on you. Why don't you run on back to the hotel and rest a bit? We'll take care of your wife. Don't you worry."

"But what will you do? Surely no more drugs," he said wearily.

"You just run along. We'll tie her to the bed, and when she finds she can't move, she'll stop all this."

He stood by my bedside listening to these words. He looked at me—his wife, his friend, his lover—and with tears streaming, he said to the nurse, "Oh, no, you will never tie down my Jean. I will lay my body on top of hers and she will recognize me and she will rest."

The nurse, her mouth agape and her eyes wide, was horrified. When she found her voice, she stammered, "What are you saying? You absolutely *cannot* even lie in her bed, much less lie on top of her! Why, you'll pull the rest of the tubes out, and besides, the whole thing is against hospital rules." She shook, she was so shocked, as she added, "You cannot do any such thing!"

My husband, this man who understood intimacy and love, stood, all six feet, three inches of him, looked that nurse straight in the eye and said, almost in a whisper, "Oh, no, not to my Jean. I *can* do this and I *will* do this." And he *did* do this and I, recognizing him, found peace in the recognition. I let go. I slept. Such power there is in love.

Jean Brody

Encounter with a God

I stand by the bed where a young woman lies, her face postoperative, her mouth twisted in palsy, clownish. A tiny twig of the facial nerve, the one to the muscles of her mouth, has been severed. She will be thus from now on. The surgeon had followed with religious fervor the curve of her flesh, I promise you that. Nevertheless, to remove the tumor in her cheek, I had to cut the little nerve.

Her young husband is in the room. He stands on the opposite side of the bed, and together they seem to dwell in the evening lamplight, isolated from me, private. *Who are they,* I ask myself, *he and this wry-mouth I have made, who gaze at and touch each other so generously, greedily?* The young woman speaks.

"Will my mouth always be like this?" she asks.

"Yes," I say, "it will. It is because the nerve was cut."

She nods and is silent. But the young man smiles.

"I like it," he says. "It is kind of cute."

All at once I *know* who he is. I understand, and I lower my gaze. One is not bold in an encounter with a god. Unmindful, he bends to kiss her crooked mouth, and I am so close I can see how he twists his own lips to accommodate hers, to show her that their kiss still works.

I remember that the gods appeared in ancient Greece as mortals, and I hold my breath and let the wonder in.

Richard Selzer, M.D.

Holding Hands

My husband Paul's hands had a fine, firm feeling: warm, never cold, never moist, their slight pressure always reassuring. And whenever those hands sought mine in the final days of his life, he pressed them both together around one of my hands.

It was during that time, as I sat by his bed, that I tried to memorize his hands. They were twice as long as mine and half a hand wider. His fingers did not taper; they were long and square, laced with fine veins all the way to the tips. His nails squared off the ends of his fingers, with clearly defined moons at the cuticles and clearly defined white edges. He had always taken great care to keep them neat. They were not tough hands nor soft, either. They were the hands of a college professor whose tools were chalk and felt-tipped red pens.

I wondered if his students had difficulty reading his hieroglyphics. I had grown used to them the year we were apart—engaged to be married, but separated—so he could pursue a master's degree at Bradley University, 800 miles away from our Pennsylvania hometown.

Had I remembered to tell him that I found his large

hands beautiful? Did I ever explain that, in our years of courtship, when he was invited regularly to dinner in my home, my mother was fascinated with the quiet way he managed the silverware and coffee cups in hands in which they nearly disappeared? Did I mention that in his clasp— in a movie, in poignant moments in church, in the hospital beds to which the illnesses of his last four years confined him—I felt pure and honest expressions of his love?

In those hands, also, originated his caring for his children. It was a point of pride that he gave our newborn daughter her first bath. At seven pounds and fourteen ounces, she fit comfortably into the length of those two hands, but his large fingers moved with grace and delicacy to bathe her and the five babies who followed.

Those hands, in our lean early years, gave haircuts to three sons in the course of their growing up and toweled three daughters' hair dry after showers.

They manipulated suitcases, with a maximum of sweat and a minimum of profanity, in top-of-the-car carriers of station wagons for twenty-eight annual summer pilgrimages to Pennsylvania to visit grandparents. They distributed Communion in church—a most honored and honorable task. They traced patterns in the air as he taught his marketing students in the university in which he had studied so many years before.

Those hands clasped mine in the most frightening moments of his illnesses. They reached for mine through seven months of chemotherapy and its agonizing side effects, through the bedfast few weeks of the end of his life, when children came to visit, give service and mourn in advance what they could clearly see was the end of their father's seventy-five years.

Those hands clasped mine in the deepest, darkest moment when he whispered into the curve of my neck, "I wonder . . . how it is to die. I wonder if it hurts." I could

only give him what I believed was the sum of his life—
that he would be surrounded, uplifted, overjoyed with
the glory of God.

Finally, he was no longer able to hold my hands. Early
one morning, I prepared Paul for the priest who had come
every day for the past week to give him a fragment of
Communion on a teaspoonful of water and bless him.
After offering Paul a breakfast he could no longer eat, in a
state of nervous anxiety I clipped, filed and whitened his
fingernails. There was no movement, no recognition, no
response as I laid his hands across his chest, where they
had lain uncharacteristically still for several days. Within
an hour, when the hospice nurse checked him with her
stethoscope, there was nothing left for me to do but close
his luminous green eyes and lay my hands on his for the
last time, in the quiet haven of our bedroom.

Months later, I opened the top drawer of Paul's dresser
one Sunday and reached in for one of his clean, pressed
handkerchiefs—I liked to use them now. What I touched
was an opened pack of emery boards.

For seven-and-a-half months, my grief for my husband
had been frozen within me like an icy presence that
would not yield. Then, this last Sunday of February, I was
undone by the simple presence of emery boards. Tears
came as I closed my eyes and tried in vain to remember
the clasp of Paul's hands.

Soon after, Stephen, the youngest—who most resembles
his father—came to see me. When it was time to go, Stephen
kissed me good-bye and then, impulsively, took my hand in
both of his large, broad ones. For several moments, I
couldn't speak. It was as though his father's long, graceful
hands clasped mine once again. Still reassuring me.

Helen Troisi Arney

5

ON
MOTHERHOOD

*God sent children for another purpose
than merely to keep up the race—
to enlarge our hearts; and to make us
unselfish and full of kindly sympathies
and affections; to give our souls higher
aims; to call out all our faculties to
extended enterprise and exertion; and
to sing round our firesides bright faces,
happy smiles and loving, tender hearts.*

Mary Botham Howitt

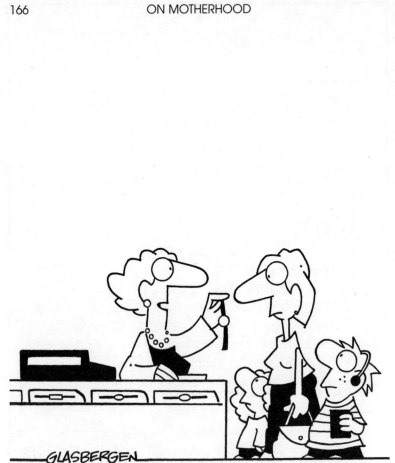

"This is the perfect watch for mothers.
Every day is thirty-six hours."

Second Skin

I looked on child rearing not only as a work of love and duty but as a profession that was fully as interesting and challenging as any honorable profession in the world, and one that demanded the best I could bring to it.

Rose Kennedy

My favorite pair of old jeans will never fit me again. I have finally accepted this immutable truth. After nurturing and giving birth to two babies, my body has undergone a metamorphosis. I may have returned to my pre-baby weight, but subtle shifts and expansions have taken place—my own version of continental drift. As a teenager, I never understood the difference between junior and misses sizing; misses clothing just looked old. Now it is all too clear that wasp waists and micro-fannies are but the fleeting trappings of youth. But that's okay, because while the jeans no longer button, the life I exchanged for them fits better than they ever did.

For me, this is a barefoot, shorts and T-shirt time of life. I have slipped so easily into young motherhood; it is the most comfortable role I have ever worn. No tough seams, no snagging zippers. Just a feeling that I have stepped out of the dressing room in something that finally feels right.

I love the feel of this baby on my hip, his soft head a perfect fit under my chin, his tiny hands splayed out like small pink starfish against my arms. I love the way my eight-year-old daughter walks alongside us as we cross the grocery store's sunny parking lot. On gorgeous spring days, the breeze lifts her wispy ponytail, and we laugh at how the sunshine makes the baby sniff and squint. I am constantly reaching out to touch them, the way a seamstress would two lengths of perfect silk, envisioning what might be made from them, yet hesitant to alter them, to lose the weight of their wholeness in my hands.

On those rare mornings when I wake up before they do, I go into their rooms and watch them sleeping, their faces creased and rosy. Finally, they squirm and stretch themselves awake, reaching out for a hug. I gather them up, bury my face in them and breathe deeply. They are like towels just pulled from the dryer, tumbled warm and cottony.

Sometimes, I follow the sound of girlish voices to my daughter's room, where she and her friends play dress-up, knee-deep in garage-sale chiffon, trying life on for size. Fussing and preening in front of the mirror, they drape themselves in cheap beads and adjust tiaras made of sequins and cardboard. I watch these little girls with their lank, shiny hair that no rubber bands or barrettes seem able to tame. They are constantly pushing errant strands behind their ears, and in that grown-up gesture, I see glimpses of the women they will become. I know that too soon these clouds of organdy and lace will settle permanently into their battered boxes, the ones that have served as treasure chests and princess thrones. They will become the hand-me-downs of my daughter's girlhood, handed back to me.

For now, though, my children curl around me on the sofa in the evening, often falling asleep, limbs limp and soft against me like the folds of a well-worn nightgown. For now, we still adorn each other, and they are content to be clothed in my embrace. I know there will be times that will wear like scratchy wool sweaters and four-inch heels. We will have to try on new looks together, tugging and scrunching, trying to keep the basic fabric intact. By then, we will have woven a complicated tapestry with its own peculiar pattern, its snags and pulls and tears.

But I will not forget *this* time, of drowsy heads against my shoulder, of footy pajamas and mother-daughter dresses, of small hands clasped in mine. *This* time fits me. I plan to wear it well.

Caroline Castle Hicks

Ron

Ron was a fifteen-year-old teenager, a tenth-grade student at Granger High School. It was game day, and he was the only sophomore suiting up with the varsity team. Excitedly, he invited his mother to attend. It was her very first football game, and she promised to be there with several of her friends. The game finally ended, and she was waiting outside the locker room to drive Ron home.

"What did you think of the game, Mom? Did you see the three touchdown passes our team made and our tough defense, and the fumble on the kickoff return that we recovered?" he asked.

His mother replied, "Ron, you were magnificent. You have such presence, and I was proud of the pride you took in the way you looked. You pulled up your knee socks eleven times during the game, and I could tell you were perspiring in all those bulky pads because you got eight drinks and splashed water on your face twice. I really like how you went out of you way to pat number nineteen, number five and number ninety on the back every time they came off the field."

"Mom, how do you know all that? And how can you

say I was magnificent? I didn't even play in the game."

His mother smiled and hugged him. "Ron, I don't know anything about football. I didn't come here to watch the game. I came here to watch you!"

Dan Clark

THE FAMILY CIRCUS   **By Bil Keane**

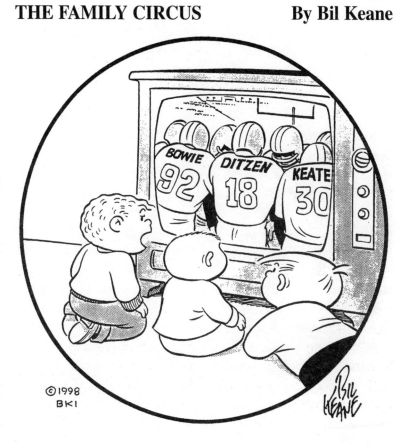

"Their mommies write their names on their shirts so they won't lose them."

Reprinted by permission of Bil Keane.

Parental Justice

Many people know me as Whoopi Goldberg, the comedienne, but few know my work—what I've gone through—as Whoopi Goldberg, the mother.

One night when my daughter was maybe thirteen or fourteen, she came downstairs and told me she was going out, and it was none of my business where. I looked this child over, this little version of me. She was wearing three pieces of cloth. The cloth itself was all shiny and nice and fine, but it wasn't covering enough to suit a mother. It wasn't even close. It was probably against the law, in some states, to go out looking like she wanted to go out looking. Okay, in my time I wore a mini so small that all I needed to do was sneeze and you would have known exactly what color my panties were, but here was my barely teenage daughter, looking like a grown woman, dressed like Madonna used to dress. I completely flipped.

Before my mother could come out of my mouth, she was in my ear. I heard her chuckling in the corner, laughing at me over the way our situation had turned. This was parental justice. Her laugh took me back, and I got angry.

"Why are you laughing?" I shot back.

"Because it's funny," she said. "Because it's funny to see you like this now."

Funny? I'm trying to explain to this child that she can't go out looking like this. She can't go out looking like this because you don't know what invitation someone is going to pick up from this.

That line—*you don't know what invitation someone is going to pick up from this*—was one of my mother's, and I wanted to take it right back as soon as I'd said it. My mother looked over at me and smiled, and at first I tried not to smile back, but it was too late. I had to smile too. It wasn't one of those let-me-laugh-along-with-you kind of smiles, or one of those gee-ain't-we-funny kind of smiles, but the kind of smile that comes from knowing.

I got it. Finally. I understood. It was a smile of recognition, and maybe a little surrender. I reconnected to everything that passed between us, and I could see what was coming. I wanted to tell my mother how sorry I was for putting her through all of those motions, for not recognizing that she had something to offer beyond what I could see. But she knew. She smiled back and she knew.

I turned to my kid and said, "You know what? Go out. Just go."

And she did. She looked at me funny—suspicious—but she went out like she had planned. And then she came back, about twenty minutes later. "You know what?" she said. "It's cold out there. I think I'm going to change, put a little more on."

It happens, but it takes time. I watch now as my daughter goes through it for herself, with her own kids, and I try not to chuckle. I know someday she'll hear me coming out of her mouth and she'll look over with one of those knowing smiles and start to laugh, because we all get it, eventually.

Whoopi Goldberg

DENNIS THE MENACE

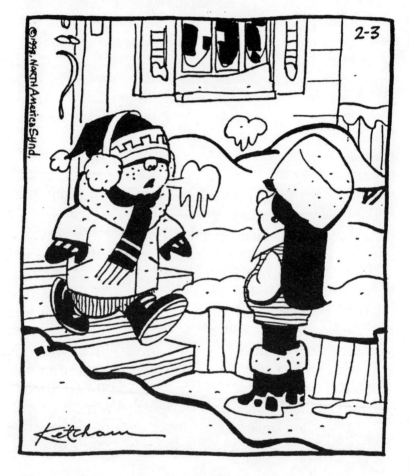

"Staying bundled up makes my mom feel warm
all over."

Ry

At his request, each morning three-year-old Ry's mother pinned a bath towel to the back shoulders of his size two T-shirt. Immediately in his young imaginative mind, the towel became a brilliant magic blue and red cape. And he became Superman.

Outfitted each day in his "cape," Ry's days were packed with adventure and daring escapades. He was Superman.

This fact was clearly pointed out last fall when his mother enrolled him in kindergarten class. During the course of the interview, the teacher asked Ry his name.

"Superman," he answered politely and without pause.

The teacher smiled forgivingly, cast an appreciative glance at his mother, and asked again, "Your real name, please."

Again, Ry answered, "Superman."

Realizing the situation demanded more authority, or maybe to hide amusement, the teacher closed her eyes for a moment, then in a voice quite stern, said, "I will have to have your real name for the records."

Sensing he'd have to play straight with the teacher, Ry

slid his eyes around the room, hunched closer to her, and patting a corner of frayed towel at his shoulder, answered in a voice hushed with conspiracy: "Clark Kent."

Joyce Meier

Finding a Son

I felt like I was giving birth again as I walked into the adoption agency to meet my grown son. The physical pain was absent this time, but the anxiety was just as high. It had been almost a quarter of a century since that scared and lonely girl had last seen her firstborn child.

I didn't remember much about that young girl anymore. Over the years, new experiences and tragedies had taken over the rooms where those memories had lived. The feelings that had survived weren't clear either; they had all run together, producing a dull ache that never let up.

Twenty-five years ago, my boyfriend and I had lived without thought for how our actions would impact the future. Morning sickness was my wake-up call. Though we had been carefree, the laws weren't, and at that time, ending a pregnancy could have meant ending my life, too. I had no choice but to confront my fear and my parents. It would be painful, but it wouldn't be fatal.

Everyone cried and took a slice of responsibility. I took the biggest piece because I was eating for two—the absent father and myself. Fortunately, I gained weight slowly—slow enough to be undetected by outsiders, and more important, by my younger brother. My mother shied away from explaining my condition to him, so I dutifully camouflaged myself. I didn't want to be sent away.

My mother and I passed the next few months like ladies of leisure. We shopped, we redecorated, and we lunched. I was a little girl again, home with the flu and being entertained by my mommy so I wouldn't dwell on how bad I felt.

The tactic worked in the daylight hours, but at night in my bed, I faced the cold truth. I wouldn't wake to find that my pregnancy had broken in the night like a fever. In fact, each day brought increased physical awareness that I was not alone in my body. It began with a flutter that could have been too much pizza, but within a few days, I knew this was not a bodily function. This little being was becoming real to me. I yearned to share the excitement of this discovery with someone, but there was only my mother, and I didn't want to hurt her. I felt that I could revel in this experience now and still do what was expected of me later. But I knew that this first-time grandmother would find it hard to face the fact that she would allow herself to hand her newborn grandchild to strangers.

The soft rumblings that had lulled me to sleep now became urgent jabs. My nights were increasingly sleepless, and my days were filled with backaches and boredom. I had to discontinue all projects that required lifting, bending or climbing, and I couldn't go out anymore because someone might recognize me. Eventually, this started to get to me, and I felt that unless I was ready to have my baby on the psychiatric floor of the hospital, I had to get out for a while. A girlfriend suggested we go to a new club, and suddenly, I was an eighteen-year-old girl again. "What are you going to wear?" took on a whole new meaning. Fortunately, Empire dresses were the fashion and hid my seven-month stomach.

At the club, I found it frightening being out among people my own age again, especially in my condition. But as we settled into seats away from the dance floor, I began to relax and enjoy the new sound called disco. I pretended that it was a year ago, and I hadn't yet messed up my life.

Suddenly, I was brought back to reality by a young man's face peering into mine and asking me to dance. I hadn't planned on this, but maybe if I didn't move too fast, no one would guess. I was concentrating on my balance and the new dance steps when the disc jockey started a slow song. All the breath seemed to rush out of me as my partner took hold of my hand and prepared to slide his arm around my waist. There was no time to pull away; in a second, this cute college boy would realize he'd been flirting with a pregnant woman. Would he drop his arms with a look of revulsion and leave me alone on the light-speckled platform? But wait, we were still dancing. Could it be he hadn't noticed I was leaning like a bell? Then, as I was congratulating myself for being so controlled, someone close to me woke up.

The movement started small—like a cat stretch, and I silently pleaded, *Go back to sleep baby,* but he wanted to dance, too. The song was almost over, and it looked as if my luck would hold—until my little partner tried a new dance move. Before I could lean away, a tiny foot shot against my abdomen. I cautiously glanced up, and my big partner was smiling. Did that mean it was okay that someone else's child was kickboxing his body?

"You must be real hungry; even I felt that rumble," he said as the music finally stopped.

I would need that amusing memory to get through the next few weeks. Everything that had been physically uncomfortable became worse. It would be happening soon. I would be ripped apart. All the falling out of trees and off bikes would not equal this one excruciating day of pain.

As I came to in the recovery room, it wasn't the contractions and delivery that left me hurting. I can still see the nurse's face, telling me to stop crying. "You'll just have to live with it!" she said. In her cruel way, she was prophetic. I *did* live with it; through the ten minutes they allowed me to hold my son in my arms and the following nine thousand days I would hold him in my heart alone.

One afternoon, decades of living later, my therapist, in a moment of inspiration, said, "Okay, you can't change a lot of what's happened, but you can finish this chapter. Go find your son."

So I had. And now I was walking past the offices and down the stairs toward the room where he waited. I had taken such care getting ready, and although I looked mature, inwardly I didn't feel like the mother of a twenty-four-year-old man. I was that frightened girl again, imagining that the workers in the offices upstairs were making unflattering remarks about me. The counselor took my arm to steady me as we entered the room.

"This is your son," he said, and to him: "and this is your mother. Take all the time you want."

By the time he had finished speaking, I had covered the remaining distance and was being embraced by a tall, dark and handsome young man. I pulled away just enough to study his face, a familiar face. I had looked at that face many times in a portrait on my mother's dresser—only there, the face wore a World War II army cap. This child I had tried so hard to visualize had grown into the image of my father. We hugged and kissed, laughed, cried, asked and answered questions for well over ten minutes.

All the people in the offices upstairs were smiling, and some were wiping their eyes as we walked out hand in hand.

That was three years ago, and since then, many of my family members have been introduced to my newfound son: his sister and two brothers, and my own little brother—the uncle who had been an adult before he knew I'd had a fourth child. My first son finally met his grandfather, giving my father the rare opportunity of seeing himself as he was fifty years ago. My mother would never meet her first grandchild, as she had passed away eight years before I made the decision to find my son.

For me, it had been the right decision. I felt so fortunate that we found each other, and that we felt so comfortable together. I didn't think there could be more, but I was wrong.

Five months ago, my firstborn and his lovely wife completed this circle of life. My son handed me his son, and I cried with joy that the next nine thousand days would be ours to share.

Lin Faubel

Snowballs and Lilacs

What would I want engraved on my grave-stone for posterity? "Mother."

Jessica Lange

I set the big, manila envelope on my mother's table, continuing our ordinary conversation, trying to draw away from the importance of this package and its contents. Through sentences of chit-chat, I worked up the courage from within, until I finally asked her to open it. She did, with a Norwegian sparkle in her blue eyes, expecting a surprise. She grew quiet as she pulled out the picture inside, and saw my own dark brown eyes staring back at her in the face of another woman. The resemblance was startling, and realization swept across her face as she turned to me with joy and wonder and whispered, "Is this your *real* mother?"

Biting my lip, a trick I had learned from her to hold back the tears, I realized this wonderful woman of substance in front of me had never seemed more precious than at this moment. A flash of all the years she had spent caring for my brothers and me flickered through my mind, as well as the life she led—a life that knew no other way than to put her children and others first on a daily basis. With the knowledge of what was truly "real," I answered her with borrowed wisdom and responded, "Yes, it's a picture of my birth mother."

My search for her had been a need for self-fulfillment, to answer all those nagging questions once wondered. My inquiry had brought feelings of guilt as well. Although my parents had always encouraged me to look, saying that they were just as curious, I didn't want either one of them to be hurt in the process, or to think that I loved them any less. I secretly marveled at their encouragement, and the confidence that it represented in my steadfast love for them. But after a lifetime of unconditional love and bonding, they had well earned that security.

My mother's eyes saddened as I told her that my birth mother had died; both my mother and I had often hoped for the day when we would be able to thank her personally. Now that connection would never come.

On Memorial Day, I took my two young sons to the cemetery to place flowers on my birth mother's grave. We first stopped at the gravesides of my grandparents. My mother had obviously been there, having left her home-made bouquet of snowballs and lilacs—an annual tradition of hers. Year after year, I had found comfort in those flowers, always there, loved ones always remembered. They reminded me of my mother in their simple but God-given beauty. I smiled as I thought of the daffodils she gave me each birthday—one for each year of my life. When I was younger, Mom's time-honored yellow tradition had been taken for granted. Now at the age of thirty-five, I counted each one, each flower so significant. Nothing would make me happier than to adopt a little girl and continue that tradition with her.

But now was not the time to be a daughter dabbling in

daydreams, but to be a mother myself. My sons tugged on my hands, playing tug-of-war with my thoughts. We hurried off to our last stop, my birth mother's grave. Our pace slowed as we neared the general location, and we solemnly walked through row after row of beautifully decorated tombstones. I knew we were looking for a plain simple stone, without flowers.

I had formed friendships in the last several months with my birth sisters and brother. Although they deeply loved my birth mother, I knew they were not ones to visit cemeteries. Somehow that made it even more important that I come. She definitely deserved flowers, to be remembered, and so very much more. But after half an hour of searching unsuccessfully, my sons were growing impatient, so I decided I would have to come back by myself. We were just about to leave when I spotted it.

Not her name. Not an empty stone. But the same simple bouquet of snowballs and lilacs that I had seen earlier, the ones most assuredly that had been placed there by my mother. Mom had already been there, in the morning's early hours, to show her gratitude and the respect she felt for the importance of this woman's life, and the great gift she had given.

As I knelt and closely looked at the dates, I noticed the epitaph, which so appropriately read, "Beloved Mother." Biting my lip, I couldn't hold back the tears as I honored this remarkable woman who had given me life, and my own beloved mother, who had given that life such meaning.

Lisa Marie Finley

The Little Princess

My nine-year-old daughter, Vivien, is a little princess, who under normal circumstances can't even pour herself a glass of milk. Even as a baby, she had such a regal air that her father and I used to joke that she must have discovered us under the heading "slaves" in some catalog for pre-womb babies searching for parents.

Now that I'm a single parent, I'm her only attendant-in-waiting during her time with me. So when I came home shivering with fever at lunchtime one day last week, my first thought was, *How will Her Royal Littleness react?* It would be too much to expect her to actually leave me in peace to rest, much less to care for me in any way. But would she at least be willing to forage for herself at mealtime?

At 3:30 P.M., I dragged myself out of bed and drove to school to pick her up. In the car on the way home, I said, "Sweetheart, Mommy's really sick, and I've got to go to bed as soon as we get home. I'm sorry, but I can't do anything for you tonight. I can't make dinner, or run your bath, or anything. I've just got to rest. Do you think you could manage to fix your own meal tonight?"

"That's okay," she replied unconcernedly, but this didn't reassure me. The real test would come when she actually wanted something.

When we arrived home, I crawled back upstairs to bed, where I lay, miraculously undisturbed, for the next six hours. Well, almost undisturbed. Every now and then, I would wake from a feverish sleep to find a little angel bending over me with some goodwill offering. A cool, wet washcloth to wipe my hot brow. A brass bell to ring if I wanted anything. A picture she had drawn to cheer me up of a kitten basking in the sun. A "feel-good," pink bow-tied teddy bear that someone had brought her once when she was sick, and in whose medicinal properties she seemed to place great faith.

During one of her visitations, I announced that I needed to go downstairs to the bathroom. Vivien solicitously helped me on with my sweater "in order to keep you warm," and she insisted on my leaning on her—all four feet of her—in order to negotiate the stairs. When I wandered into the kitchen and out of habit began to put dishes away, my little princess sternly interrupted me. "Mommy, you're doing too much stuff. Go back to bed." I meekly obeyed.

Throughout the evening, Vivien issued periodic reports on her progress with the evening routine. "I just made myself a salad for dinner." Or, "I'm running my bath now."

The *pièce de résistance* came at bedtime. She announced, in her best mommy-imitation voice, "I'm just going downstairs to see whether anything else needs to be done. Then I'm going to brush my teeth, turn out the lights and go to bed." I smiled to myself under the blankets.

Then Vivien produced a little book she had made for me by cutting out pieces of colored paper and stapling them together. The first page read, "I LOVE YOU MOMMY." The second page read, "You are so pretty

MOMMY!" The third page read, "Thank you for all the things you did for me MOMMY." The fourth page read, "You don't know how cool you are MOMMY." The fifth page read, "You are the Best MOMMY." The sixth page exhorted, "Good job MOMMY." The seventh page concluded, "Go MOMMY!"

I started to cry as I read this testimony of love from my daughter. Just the day before, I had been feeling overwhelmed and unappreciated as a parent. Today, not only had Vivien taken care of herself and me beautifully, she had also reassured me that I was very much loved and valued indeed. Her actions and words that day made all the things I do for her worthwhile and gave me more strength than any medicine could have. As she disappeared downstairs to close up the house for the night, I felt a wave of gratitude for the illness that had given my little princess the opportunity to demonstrate—and me the opportunity to appreciate—what a sweet and generous little angel she truly is.

Wendy Miles

When Did She Really Grow Up?

Every night after I tucked her into bed, I sang to her, a silly song, a made-up song, our song. "Stay little, stay little, little little stay; little stay little stay little."

She would giggle and I would smile. The next morning I would say: "Look at you. You grew. The song didn't work."

I sang that song for years, and every time I finished, she crossed her heart and promised she wouldn't grow any more.

Then one night, I stopped singing it. Who knows why. Maybe her door was closed. Maybe she was studying. Maybe she was on the phone talking to someone. Or maybe I realized it was time to give her permission to grow.

It seems to me now that our song must have had some magic because all the nights I sang it, she remained a baby... four, five, six, seven, eight, nine, ten. They felt the same. They even looked the same. She got taller and her feet got bigger and some teeth fell out and new ones grew in, but she still had to be reminded to brush them and her hair and to take a shower every now and then.

She played with dolls and Play-Doh. Though Candy Land was abandoned for Monopoly and Clue, across a table, there she still was. For years, she was like those wooden dolls that nest one inside the other, identical in everything but size.

Or at least that's how I saw her. She roller-skated and ice-skated and did cartwheels in shopping malls and blew bubbles and drew pictures, which we hung on the refrigerator. She devoured Yodels and slushes and woke early on Sunday mornings to watch *Davey and Goliath*.

She never slept through the night, not at ten months, not at ten years. When she was small, she'd wake and cry and I'd take her into bed with me. When she got bigger, she'd wake and make her way down the hall, and in the morning, I would find her lying beside me.

She used to put notes under my pillow before she went to bed. I used to put notes in her bologna sandwiches before she went to school. She used to wait by the phone when I was away. I used to wait at the bus stop for her to come home.

The song, the notes, the waking up to find her next to me, the waiting at the bus stop—all these things ended a long time ago. Upstairs now is a young woman, a grown-up. She has been grown up for a while. Everyone else has seen this—everyone but me.

I look at her today, one week before she graduates from high school, and I am proud of her, proud of the person she has become. But I'm sad, too—not for her, but for me. There has been a child in this house for twenty-five years. First one grew up, then the other, but there was always this one . . . the baby.

Now the baby is grown. And despite what people tell me—*you don't lose them, they go away but they come home again, you'll like the quiet when she's gone, the next part of life is the best*—I know that what lies ahead won't be like what was.

I loved what was. I loved it when she toddled into my

office and set up her toy typewriter next to mine. I loved watching her run down the hall at nursery school straight into my arms, after a separation of just two-and-a-half hours. I loved taking her to buy stickers and for walks and to movies. I loved driving her to gymnastics and listening to her friends. I loved being the one she raced to when she was happy or frightened or sad. I loved being the center of her world.

"Mommy, come play with me."

"Mommy, I'm home."

"Mommy, I love you the bestest and the widest."

What replaces these things?

"Want to see my cap and gown?" she says now, peeking into my office. She holds it up. She smiles. She's happy. I'm happy for her. She kisses me on the cheek and says, "I love you, Mom." And then she walks upstairs.

I sit at my desk and though my heart hurts, I smile. I think what a privilege motherhood is, and how very lucky I am.

Beverly Beckham

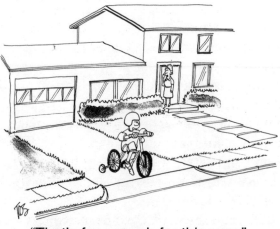

"That's far enough for this year."

Reprinted by permission of Andrew Toos.

Children on Loan

I am not good at returning things. Take library books. I have no intention of keeping them, but it takes a jolt to separate us—like a call from the librarian. Today, they sit awaiting return three days early. Because today, I'm painfully aware of the passage of time. In thirty minutes, assuming my son is packed—and he will be—Christopher Paul ("the best boy of all," he'd tease his sisters) leaves for his last year of college. He's our youngest, the last to leave home. By now, I tell myself, I am used to these departures. *I am used to these departures. I am used to these departures . . .*

Only this one is for keeps. Next May, there will be no bags of soiled laundry coming home. Chris won't be coming home at all. After graduation, it's marriage to Pam—the sunny Californian, adorable and already beloved by us all—and on to start their life together a thousand miles away. Every tick of our copper kitchen clock says, *This—is—it. Emp—ty—nest.*

My sister, the research chemist, calls. "For Pete's sake, you knew it was coming."

"So is the end of the world, but who's ready for it?"

"You really are in a mood."

My silence speaks for itself. Who knows us as well as our sisters?

"After all," she adds, "he'll be home for the holidays. Anyway, you wouldn't want to keep him forever."

My sister does not read me well at all. I find myself caressing my chunky Timex as tenderly as I would a newborn's head. We've ticked away a lot of time together— waiting outside schools, athletic fields, piano lessons, rehearsals, practices. Later, awake in bed, listening for his first car to pull into the drive. Waiting as time dragged by. Now, in take-off time, seconds spring ahead.

The doorbell summons me to a girl selling candy for her school band. The six chocolate bars are my excuse to visit Chris's room with him still in it. Boxes block the doorway. A barricade? Walls easily erect themselves at times like these. At his "Hi, Mom," I try to read his voice. Glad I'm here? Resentful of intrusion?

He's tossing items into a carton labeled MED.CAB.SUPPLIES. Glancing down on stomach soothers, skin scrubbers, lens solution, musky colognes, I'm reminded of the bottle of cheap aftershave he was so thrilled to find in his stocking one long-ago Christmas. He used it up in a week, but his room reeked all winter. "Ever try this?" he asks now, holding up a new brand of tooth gel. I smile brightly as I shake my head, but I have the ugly urge to snatch his alien brand and write TRAITOR on his suitcase. We all use Crest. We've always used Crest!

I realize my hand still clutches a damp tissue when I find myself using it to wipe his battered alarm clock. A wasted effort. Not only is it no longer smeared with peanut butter or sticky with Coke, I notice it is among the abandoned.

"This still dependable?"

"Never failed me yet."

Which means just fifteen minutes to go. "Time for a quick cup of coffee?" I would climb a Brazilian mountain and hand-pick beans to buy more time.

"Sure." He smiles in the lopsided way I love. He'll make a handsome bridegroom, but I really didn't have that in mind when I nagged him into slimming down in eighth grade.

It's been a long time since I stood watching coffee perk. I remember putting his early bottle on to warm, then starting the coffee. We snuggled cheek to cheek, waiting for our morning brews. He was warm with baby-sleep, I with mother-love. Neither of us minded the wait.

Now, sitting across from Chris as I gulp from my hot mug, I have to content myself with coffee and conversation. As appreciative as I am for our small talk, I'm aware of resenting it. More meaningful words could be said. I see by his watch that it's time for him to go. His hands are exactly like my father's. Odd I never noticed before. What else have I missed?

His eyes grow sober as he begins to speak of yesterday and seeing Pam off to her college, how they worked at keeping it light. I detect a message here for me, too. God knows I'm trying. And I wouldn't mind a little help from the Man Upstairs right now. *You got me into this,* I tell him. *You let me share in your birthing business, but you messed up on the motherhood bit—or else I didn't read the fine print at the end.*

"Well . . . " Chris stands and shoves in his chair. Never once has he shoved in his chair. "Now it's *This is it, old chair. So long, old kitchen, old mother . . . "*

I stand, too, but let my chair be. He bends over and gives me a kiss. It's always a sweet surprise, the firm kiss that shows he's not afraid of affection between us. Does he know how much it means?

"Hey . . . I'll call once I'm settled," he says, and his

sensitivity triggers my tears.

"I really am trying to keep it light," I choke out with a tight laugh.

"Mom, it isn't as though . . . "

"I know. I know."

Three minutes A.D.—After Departure—I've blown my nose, repaired my make-up and am armed with my books. As I head for the door, my eyes happen to light on the plaque above it. It's hung there for years, overlooked as we hastily, purposefully, moved through our lives as a family. The line from Tennyson must have been waiting for just this moment.

God gives us love. Something to love, he lends us.

Children on loan. And I've never been good at returning things.

Norma R. Larson

6

MAKING A DIFFERENCE

*Spread love everywhere you go: first of all
in your own house . . . let no one ever come
to you without leaving better and happier.
Be the living expression of God's kindness;
kindness in your face, kindness in your eyes,
kindness in your warm greeting.*

Mother Teresa

Virtues

In this world we must help one another.

Jean de La Fontaine

In 1996, on a Friday in February, a fourteen-year-old boy walked into my son's junior high school, took out the gun he had hidden in his coat, and killed two students and a teacher.

Our small community was shattered. The following Monday, school was in session for students who wanted to come, and I decided to go to the school, just to be there. There were a few more mothers, some policemen and others from the community who had the same idea. We hugged kids, let them talk and cry—whatever we could do to comfort them. They were like little zombies, still in shock, full of fear and hurt. What I noticed most was an emptiness in their eyes. The innocence and enthusiasm that normally radiated from the faces of those children were gone.

I continued volunteering at the junior high for the rest of the school year. In October, the school hired me as the community resources director so I could go on working with the children at the school. Lunchroom duty was part of my job, and I made it a point to smile at the students, talk to them and laugh with them. I wanted to be a positive force in a place that was threatening to sink under the weight of negative emotions.

Then right before Christmas break, only ten months after the first shooting, the unthinkable happened. Another boy from the junior high went home and shot his sister, his mother and himself. The community was utterly devastated. The fragile confidence we had worked so hard to build was destroyed. Our entire community was numb with grief. The emptiness I had seen in the children's eyes spread to the adults as well. I didn't know if we would be able to recover.

Over the holidays, I wept and prayed. I have always found comfort and inspiration in prayer, and during that dark time, an idea came to me. I wanted to do something to fill the emptiness I saw all around me. What if everyone, the whole town, focused on virtues? The idea was very specific and yet simple. First, get everyone thinking about virtues. Then, start encouraging everyone to look for the virtues in their lives—in others and in themselves. Next and most important, teach people to acknowledge the virtues they saw around them. I didn't know if it would work, but I knew I had to try.

I decided to start with four virtues: compassion, respect, responsibility and tolerance. I had 150 signs made—the virtues and their definitions in bold black lettering on white sheets. My plan was to put up the signs at school and then have the children help me put more signs in all the local store windows. I wanted to flood the community with something positive, to raise community awareness of what was important—what was ultimately true—in life.

I was afire with my idea. The principal of the junior high was supportive of the plan, so I jumped into the program my son and I named "Virtuous Reality." I immediately met with resistance from some of the students. There was one student named Andy who was the ringleader of the kids who were "too cool" for the virtues program. Andy definitely had an attitude: He was sullen, sarcastic and rude, the epitome of the defiant teenager. I knew I had to win him over if I was going to get anywhere with my plan. So I kept Andy in my prayers.

One weekend, I had an inspiration about Andy. Again, my idea was very clear and specific. I was so excited, I wasn't sure that I could wait for Monday to try it out.

Monday morning, when I walked into the school office, Andy was sitting outside the principal's office. He had been sent there to "discuss" the safety pin he was sporting through his ear. He was in a surly mood and almost snarled at me as I walked by him.

I sat down at my desk and called to him "Andy, come over here."

He looked up and grimaced, but he got up and shuffled reluctantly over to my desk. "Yeah, what do you want?" he said sourly.

"I was thinking about you this weekend," I told him.

He was astonished. "You were?" he said, the tough-guy mask slipping a little.

"Yes, I was," I said. "Do you like animals?"

"Yeah," he said cautiously.

"Especially dogs?"

"Yeah. How did you know that?" By now, he was simply a curious fourteen-year-old boy. It was working.

Ignoring his question, I continued, "Do you know what it takes to be an animal lover?" He shook his head no. "It takes compassion."

Immediately, I saw his shoulders relax and his face soften. "Andy," I continued, "you are a man of compassion. Did you know that?"

"No," he said in a small voice. His face was so sweet, it

was hard to believe he was the same child.

I kept going. "Do you let that side of you show to your friends?" When he shook his head no, I said, "People are really attracted to compassion, Andy. If you showed that side of you to people, they'd be attracted to you for all the right reasons."

We ended our conversation with a pinky promise, which if you know teenage boys, is an indication of how melted this guy was. I made him link pinkies with me and promise to show his compassion to others for the coming week.

After that, Andy was on my side. We had connected deeply. He knew that I saw—and more important, acknowledged—the good in him.

Since then, the virtues program has flourished. The students love it, and it has become a community project as well. Every week, the students pick one virtue for the whole town to focus on. There are signs up in school and all over town. Students discuss the week's virtue in classes, and even the radio stations feature "Virtuous Reality" spots throughout the week. Recently, in the local hospital, we've created a virtue wall. Students take one virtue, illustrate it quilt-block style, and then a local artist transposes it onto the wall at the hospital. Feelings of love and hope are steadily replacing our emptiness.

Certainly, the tragedies we experienced changed our little community forever. But some of those changes have been major transformations. Last week, while attending a pep rally at the high school, I was amazed to see Andy, now a sophomore, dancing in front of the whole student body with the drill team. Afterwards, as I was standing in the hall, Andy ran up to me, his face alight with joy. "Mrs. T!" he yelled. Then he gave me a big hug. "Compassion!" he whooped. Then he was off again down the hall.

Colleen Trefz

[EDITORS' NOTE: *For more information about the Virtuous Reality program and how it could impact your community, contact Colleen Trefz at 509-766-7291.*]

Sharing

Just home from work, Daddy stopped in the kitchen where Mother was cooking supper and I was setting the table. From the look on his face, we knew something was bothering him.

"Charles Roth's father is worse," he said. "The doctor says it's only a matter of time now. The old man doesn't complain much about his pain, only about the long hours he has to spend alone. His eyes are so bad he can't read, and he doesn't get much company. He keeps begging for a big dog to be his companion, one he can reach out and touch as he sits in his wheelchair in the sun."

"Why don't they buy him a dog?" I asked.

"Honey, with Mr. Roth in the hospital so much of the time, there are a lot of expenses. There isn't enough money."

"They could go to the animal shelter and get one," I suggested.

"Yes," Daddy said. "I suppose they could. But it has to be a special dog, one they can trust to be gentle. Not all big dogs are."

After supper, I went out back where my big German

shepherd, Dan, was dozing under a tree. He sprang up and ran to meet me as he always did when I came into sight. There were no other twelve-year-old girls in our neighborhood, so I depended on Dan for companionship. When I rode my bicycle, he ran behind me; when I roller-skated on the sidewalk, he trotted behind. It had been that way since Daddy brought him home, a fat brown puppy, four years before.

Now, I couldn't forget Daddy's words in the kitchen. I threw my arms around Dan's neck and buried my face in his stiff hair. He sensed my unhappiness and started whining.

"I love you," I whispered to him. "I'd be lost without you, but . . . oh, Dan, I know what I should do, but I don't want to do it."

I thought about Mr. Roth. He was old, sick and almost blind. It seemed to me that he was just about out of blessings. I got up quickly. I knew what I had to do, and if I didn't do it right now, I'd talk myself out of it.

I found Daddy sitting in his big chair, looking at his newspaper. Although we weren't supposed to interrupt him when he was reading, I blurted out, "Dan can go."

He looked over the top of the paper at me. "What did you say?" he asked.

"Mr. Roth can borrow Dan." Tears started down my face.

Daddy pitched his newspaper over the arm of the chair to the floor. "Come here," he said, reaching out for me. I crawled, long legs and all, into his lap and his arms encircled me.

"I don't really want him to go," I whimpered. "I'll miss him terribly. But Daddy, it's what I ought to do, isn't it?"

"It's what I'd be very proud to see you do," he said.

"They'll be good to him, won't they?" I asked.

"They will take good care of Dan," he assured me softly.

"The yard has a high fence, and Charles's father will be

out there in his wheelchair with him most of the time. I'll ask Charles to chain Dan when he's in the yard alone so he can't jump the fence and get lost."

I didn't like to think of Dan fenced in or chained. He and I ran free together. He'd hate being restricted. And he'd hate being away from me. How were we going to manage without each other?

As though he read my thoughts, Daddy said, "It won't be for too long, honey. Remember what the doctor said about Mr. Roth?"

I got up quickly. I couldn't talk about it anymore.

"Please call him," I said tightly. "Tell him to come and get Dan tonight." My voice wavered and I added, "Before I change my mind."

I was drying supper dishes when Charles Roth and his wife arrived. They promised me they would take good care of Dan and told me I was making a sick old man very happy.

When I tried to go to sleep that night, all I could think of was my Dan, on the other side of the city, across the river, at least ten or twelve miles away.

The next afternoon, I floundered about unhappily. My older sister, Leila, had a girlfriend over, and they didn't want a kid sister hanging around. Riding my bike or skating alone was no fun. Feeling sorry for myself, I got a book and sat under the tree to read. That's all there was to do!

The rest of the week dragged by somehow, and the next one followed. On Saturday, when I finished my chore of dusting the dining room chairs—even the bottom rungs that Mother always inspected—I volunteered to dust the living room for Leila, just to have something to do.

After lunch, it was my turn to take the scraps out to the garbage can. As I swung the screen door open and stepped out on the back porch, a big brown dog ran up the steps, his long tongue hanging out. He jumped against me, his paws on my shoulders, his eyes on my face.

"Dad, Mother!" I cried. "Leila, come here quick. Look! Dan's home!"

From inside the kitchen, Mother called, "The front doorbell is ringing. I'll answer it." And then Mother called for Daddy. I heard her say, "Charles Roth is here."

I bent down to gather my dog in my arms. He licked my arms and rubbed his head hard against my chin. I filled his bowl with water from the yard faucet and knelt beside him, stroking his back while he lapped hungrily at the water. Once or twice, he paused long enough to lick my arm, but he returned quickly to his drinking. He must have been very thirsty.

Daddy and Charles Roth came out onto the back porch.

"Well, I see him," Mr. Roth exclaimed, "but I still can't believe it!"

Early that morning, Charles Roth had rolled his father's wheelchair into the backyard and unfastened the chain from Dan's collar so that the old man could pet him and play fetch with him. Later, old Mr. Roth was wheeled back into the house while Charles and his wife went grocery shopping.

"I was in a rush and didn't remember to chain the dog. And I suppose he was smart enough to realize he was alone and free to jump the fence and come home."

While he talked, I looked at my dog. It was amazing that he found his way back. He had been taken by car at night to the Roths' home, a place he'd never seen before. There was no way he could have seen the streets and figured out a return route. How had he done it?

Mr. Roth answered my question with his next words. "It was pure love that directed that dog's path back to you," he told me. "And as hard as it will be for me to tell my father he won't be back, I can't ask you to let me take him from you again."

I looked at Daddy and his face told me he wouldn't ask

it either. I looked at Dan, stretched full length on the back-yard grass. He was completely relaxed, totally happy to be home. And I was so happy to have him back!

But then I remembered the old man in his wheelchair. He was going to be sad, his happy days with a dog over. He would be lonely again, the way I was lonely when Dan was gone.

The way I was lonely. . . . Only it wouldn't be like that because I was not sick or old, and I didn't have to sit in a wheelchair all the time. I could do lots of things. I could ride my bike and skate, even without Dan there. And I could read; old Mr. Roth couldn't do that.

"Mr. Roth," I said on impulse, "I want you to take Dan back with you."

Both he and Daddy looked at me in surprise, but I grinned at them, saying, "On one condition. You have to promise to let me come and visit him. Maybe Dan won't try to come home if he knows he'll see me soon."

I looked at Daddy. "Maybe once a week you or Mother would take me over in the car and let me spend the after-noon. I could see Dan. And I could read to Mr. Roth if he wanted me to."

That's how I began spending every Thursday afternoon with old Mr. Roth. He remembered some wonderful books from his childhood—books I might never have dis-covered on my own—and we enjoyed them together. Between our visits, he thought up riddles to ask me, and I baked cookies to take for our backyard picnics. We grew to love each other dearly, and Charles Roth said Dan and I made the old man's last days happy.

Dan was always glad to see me, and he whined a little some days when I left. But he never tried to come home again, until three months later . . . after old Mr. Roth died, when we brought him in our car to be with me for the rest of his life.

I loved Dan more than any dog I've ever had. He was smart and loyal and he loved me so completely. But more than that, he helped me learn that the love you share is the love you keep.

Drue Duke

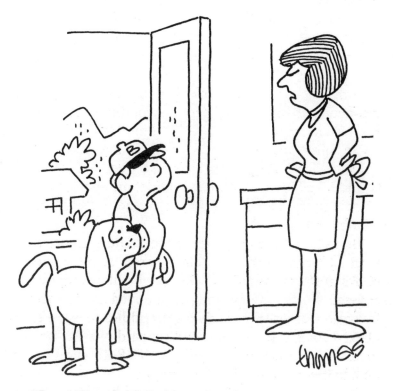

"Even if he did follow you home, you can't keep him. Send the little boy home."

Reprinted by permission of GOING BONKERS Magazine. *Please call to order at* 800-777-1999 *or online at* www.goingbonkers.com.

It's Really Christmas Now

The Sunday before Christmas last year, my husband, a police officer in Arlington, Texas, and I were just leaving for church when the phone rang. *Probably someone wanting Lee, who has already worked a lot of extra hours, to put in some more,* I thought. I looked at him and commanded, "We're going to church!"

"I'll leave in five minutes and be there in about twenty," I heard him tell the caller. I seethed, but his next words stopped me short.

"A Wish with Wings was broken into last night, and the presents are gone," he told me. "I have to go. I'll call you later." I was dumbfounded.

A Wish with Wings—Lee serves on the administrative board—is an organization in our area that grants wishes for children with devastating illnesses. Each year Wish also gives a Christmas party, where gifts are distributed. Some 170 donated gifts had been wrapped and were ready for the party, which was to be held that evening, less than nine hours away.

In a daze, I dressed our two children—Ben, just seventeen months, and five-year-old Kate—and we went to church. In between services, I told friends and the pastors about what had happened. The president of our Sunday school gave me forty dollars to buy more presents. One teacher said her class was bringing gifts to donate to another charitable organization and they would be happy to give some of them to Wish. *A dent,* I thought.

At 10:30 A.M., I phoned Lee at the Wish office. He was busy making other calls, so I packed up the kids and headed in his direction. I arrived at a barren scene. Shattered glass covered the front office where the thief had broken the door. The chill that pervaded the room was caused not only by the cold wind coming through the broken door but also by the dashed hopes of the several people who stood inside—including Pat Skaggs, the founder of Wish, and Adrena Martinez, the administrative assistant.

Looking out at the parking lot, I was startled to see a news crew from a local television station unloading a camera. Then I learned that Lee's first phone calls had been to the local radio and TV stations.

A few minutes later, a family who had heard a radio report arrived with gifts, already wrapped. Other people soon followed. One was a little boy who had brought things from his own room.

I left to get lunch for my kids and some drinks for the workers. When I got back, I found the volunteers eating pizzas that had been donated by a local pizza place. More strangers had arrived, offering gifts and labor. A glass-repair company had fixed the door and refused payment. We began to feel hope: Maybe we could still have the party!

Lee was fielding phone calls, sometimes with a receiver in each ear. Ben was fussing, so I headed home with him, hoping he could take a nap and I could find a baby-sitter.

Meanwhile, the city came alive. Two other police officers were going from church to church to spread the news. Lee told me later of a man who came directly from church, complete with coat and tie, and went to work on the floor, wrapping presents. A third officer, whose wife is a deejay for a local radio station, put on his uniform and stood outside the station collecting gifts while his wife made a plea on the air. The fire department agreed to be a drop-off point for gifts. Lee called and asked me to bring our van so it could be used to pick them up.

The clock was ticking. It was mid-afternoon, and 6:00 P.M.—the scheduled time of the party—was not far away. I couldn't find a sitter, and my son started running a fever of 103°, so I took him with me to the Wish building just long enough to trade cars with Lee.

Nothing I had ever witnessed could have prepared me for what I saw there—people lined up at the door, arms laden with gifts. One family in which the father had been laid off brought the presents from under their own tree. It was like a scene from *It's a Wonderful Life*.

Inside, Lee was still on the phone. Outside, volunteers were loading vans with wrapped gifts to be taken to the party site, an Elks lodge six miles away. By 5:50 P.M.—just before the first of the more than 100 children arrived— enough presents had been delivered to the lodge. Somehow, workers had matched up the donated items with the youngsters' wishes, so many received just what they wanted. Their faces shone with delight as they opened the packages. For some, it would be their last Christmas.

Those presents, however, were only a small portion of what came in during the day. Wish had lost 170 gifts in the robbery, but more than 1,500 had been donated! Lee decided to spend the night at the office to guard the surplus, so I packed some food and a sleeping bag and drove them down to the office. There, gifts were stacked to the ceiling, filling every available inch of space except for a small pathway that had been cleared to the back office.

Lee spent a quiet night, but the phone started ringing again at 6:30 A.M. The first caller wanted to make a donation, so Lee started to give him directions. "You'd better give me the mailing address," the caller said. "I'm in Philadelphia." The story had been picked up by the national news. Soon calls were coming from all over the country.

By midday, the Wish office was again filled with workers, this time picking up the extra gifts to take to other charitable organizations so they could distribute them before Christmas, just two days away. Pat and Adrena, whose faces had been tear-stained twenty-four hours earlier, were now filled with joy.

When Lee was interviewed for the local news, he summed up everyone's feeling: "It's really Christmas now." We had all caught the spirit—and the meaning—of the season.

Kitsy Jones

One Life at a Time

As our car slowly made its way through the crowded streets of Dhaka, Bangladesh's capital of 2 million people, I thought I knew what to expect. As leader of the American Voluntary Medical Team (AVMT), I had seen great suffering and devastation in Iraq, Nicaragua and Calcutta. But I wasn't prepared for what I saw in Bangladesh.

I traveled there with a group of AVMT doctors, nurses and other volunteers after a series of devastating cyclones hit the tiny country in 1991. More than 100,000 people had been killed, and now, because flooding had wiped out clean water and sanitation systems, thousands more were dying from diarrhea and dehydration. Children were dying from polio and tetanus, diseases nearly forgotten in the United States.

As we drove to the hospital where we were to set up a clinic, I thought I knew what we were up against: humid, scorching days, heavy rains and crowded conditions. After all, since Bangladesh became independent from Pakistan more than twenty years earlier, some 125 million people live in an area slightly smaller than the state of Wisconsin.

I glanced out the window at the street teeming with people: men talking in groups, women dressed in bright red and yellow saris, and children chasing each other, darting in between the many carts and rickshaws.

Then I looked more closely. The people were walking through raw sewage. A man stepped over a body in a doorway, just as one of the many body carts pulled up to haul it away. At a busy corner, I saw a woman standing very still, holding a small bundle, a baby. As I watched her face, she pulled her shawl back slightly, and I clearly saw her baby was dead. I suddenly thought of my own healthy children at home, and tears stung my eyes. I'd never seen anything so horrible.

The following day, I decided to ride out to Mother Teresa's orphanage in old Dhaka. A friend had asked me before I left home to visit and see what medical help they needed.

Two of the Little Sisters of the Poor greeted me at the gate and immediately led me to the infant floor. I was astonished to find 160 babies, mostly girls, squalling for attention from the few hardworking sisters.

"There are so many," I said, amazed.

"Some were given up because their parents couldn't feed them," one sister said.

"And others were abandoned because they are girls," said another. She explained that often females are aborted or killed at birth because they are considered inferior in the male-dominated culture. What little food there is must go to males.

The irony struck me hard. These baby girls were society's throwaways, yet what had I seen today? Women everywhere: working in the rice fields outside the city, herding children through crowded Dhaka, trying to earn a living by selling trinkets on the street, and here, at the orphanage, caring for the forgotten.

"A couple of the babies have serious medical problems," the sister said. "Would you like to see them?"

I followed her down a row of basket-style cribs to the tiny, sick little girls, both about two months old. One had a heart condition, the other, a severe cleft lip and palate.

"We can't do much more for them," the sister said. "Please help them. Whatever you can do will be a blessing."

I held each baby, stroking each girl's soft, dark hair and gazing into their small faces. How my heart ached for these innocent angels. What kind of a future did they face, if they had a future at all?

"I'll see what we can do," I said.

When I returned to the clinic, hundreds were waiting for treatment and much work needed to be done. I'm not a medical person, so my job is varied: I run the pharmacy, track down medicine when we run out, negotiate with local officials for equipment or transportation, and scout the patient line for critical cases.

By day's end, my head was swimming. The helpless babies' cries and the hundreds of faces on the streets and in our clinic all seemed to express the same thing—hopelessness. The thought startled me. *These people are without hope.* Even Calcutta had not seemed so bleak. *Without hope.* I repeated the words in my mind, and my heart sank. So much of what AVMT tries to do is give hope.

My inspiration was a woman who had dedicated her life to giving hope to others—my grandmother. We called her Lulu Belle, and she practically ran the Mississippi River town of Cairo, Illinois. She wasn't the mayor or a town official, but if a jobless man came to her back door, she'd call everyone she knew until she found the man work. Once, I came through her kitchen door and was startled to find a table full of strangers eating supper.

"A new family in town, Cindy," she said, as she set the

mashed potatoes on the table and headed to the stove for the gravy. "Just tryin' to give 'em a good start." I later learned the man hadn't yet found work, and Lulu Belle was making sure his family had at least one hot meal every day.

Lulu Belle had great faith, and it made her stronger than any woman I knew. Her favorite Bible verse was a simple one: "Do unto others as you would have them do unto you." She believed that if you treated people right, the way you would want to be treated, God would do the rest. So she never worried about where the job or the food would come from—she knew God would provide it.

But God seemed so far away in Bangladesh. I struggled with that thought at our morning meeting. We were set up in a clinic near Rangpur, in the northern part of the country, and our team had gathered to go over the day's schedule. At the meeting's end I told them what I tell every team: "Remember, we're here to give hope." But the words caught a little in my throat as I wondered how we would do it. Where would hope come from for these people, especially the women, so overwhelmed by disease, poverty and circumstance?

Already, 8,000 people were lined up for treatment. Scouting the line, I noticed something peculiar. All of them were men, many quite healthy. Not until I reached the end of the line did I see any women and children, and most of them looked very sick, some near death. My heart pounded as I realized what was happening. The men expected to be seen first, even if they were perfectly healthy. The women could wait.

I wondered what I should do. I remembered the woman I'd seen on the street, holding her dead baby, perhaps because she couldn't get care quickly enough. I thought of the abandoned babies in the orphanage, and anger and frustration welled up inside me.

Maybe a bit of Lulu Belle was with me as I rushed

past the line and back inside the clinic to tell the doctor in charge what was going on. He was as upset as I was.

"Well, what do you think?" he asked. "We can either see all these well men, or we can get the sick women and children up front."

"Let's do it," I said. "Let's do what we came here for."

I ran back outside and asked the interpreter to tell the men at the front to step aside. He did, and immediately I heard a disgruntled murmuring rumble through the crowd. The men were angry and the women were afraid to come forward. The interpreter repeated the announcement, and as we tried to get the crowd to move, a scuffle broke out and soon soldiers appeared, their guns strapped across their chests. They tried to restore order, but several men still pushed to the front of the line.

"Tell them no," I said to the interpreter, gathering all the courage I had. "Tell them we treat the sick women and children first or we fold up the clinic."

The men looked at me for a moment, then backed down and began letting the women forward. The fear and sadness I'd seen on the women's faces gave way to joy as they rushed to enter the clinic first. They smiled at me, grasping my hands and arms in thanks.

As one woman stretched out her hand to give me a flower, our eyes met, and I saw something incredible: hope. Now I understood. We didn't have to pull off a miracle. It was what my grandmother believed about doing unto others what was right. And out of that simple act, God had brought life-affirming hope.

Our doctors and nurses saved lives that day, and treated thousands during our two weeks in Bangladesh. When it was time to come home, I returned by way of the orphanage, to bring the two sick babies I'd seen back to the United States for treatment. On the plane home, I knew I'd have a surprise for my husband—that we would be adopting one of them, now our beautiful Bridget.

Several months later, I had the privilege of meeting with Mother Teresa about Calcutta's medical needs. In her beautifully simple way, she crystallized what I had felt in Bangladesh.

"How do you deal with the overwhelming needs, the disease, the death?" I asked.

"You look into one face," she said, her voice filled with peace, "and you continue the work." And know that God will do the rest.

Cindy Hensley McCain
As told to Gina Bridgeman

I Did My Best

To live in the hearts of those we leave behind is not to die.

Thomas Campbell

[EDITORS' NOTE: *Princess Diana was loved around the world for her humanitarian and compassionate work. Her easy rapport with people in need and her warm, understanding heart touched millions of lives. Here she describes the incident that turned the attention of the world to the cause of AIDS.*]

I had always wanted to hug people in hospital beds. A visit to an AIDS hospice in 1991, with Mrs. Bush, was a stepping stone for me. This particular man, who was so ill, started crying when I sat on his bed, and he held my hand, and I thought *Diana, do it, just do it,* and I gave him an enormous hug. It was just so touching because he clung to me and he cried. I thought, *Wonderful!*

On the other side of the room, a very young man, who I can only describe as beautiful, lying in his bed, told me he was going to die about Christmas. His friend, a man sitting in a chair by his bed, was crying his eyes out. "Why not me?" he said. I put my hand out to him and said: "It's not supposed to be easy, all this. Isn't it extraordinary, wherever I go, it's always those like you, sitting in a chair, who have to go through such hell, whereas those who accept they are going to die are calm?"

He said: "I didn't know that happened."

And I said: "Well, it does; you're not the only one. It's wonderful that you're actually by his bed. You'll learn so much from watching your friend."

He was crying and clung on to my hand, and I felt so comfortable in there. I just hated being taken away.

When I go into the Palace for a garden party or summit meeting dinner, I am a very different person. I conform to what's expected of me; but when I come to the hospice, I know when I turn my light off at night, I did my best.

Diana, Princess of Wales

Good Neighbors

One reason our family moved from our apartment in the middle of Chicago to a house in the suburbs was that we hoped to find for our daughters a true "neighborhood." To me, this meant a place where folks were more than mere acquaintances, where they shared laughs, exchanged recipes and baby-sitting, looked out for each other and were ready to share a cup of flour or a cup of tea.

So we moved in the summer of 1989, hoping we'd made the right decision.

To help allay the anxiety of so many changes for Anna, age ten, and Rachael, age seven, we'd promised them their very own dog. At the shelter, we found Lady, a full-grown mutt with the coloring of a German shepherd, one of the sweetest animals I'd ever met. It turned out that Lady not only charmed our girls, she was an instant attraction for most of the children in the neighborhood. As the girls and Lady and I walked around exploring, the local youngsters were drawn like magnets to the new dog on the block—and, consequently, started friendships with Lady's mistresses.

Things went well. There were many young families, and Anna and Rachael soon knew most of the many children.

On warm summer evenings, they all gathered outside, riding bikes, roller-skating up and down the sidewalks, playing hopscotch or jumping rope. The grownups would visit, too, and my husband and I discovered many couples with whom we had much in common.

But there was one couple who lived in a house across the street who never came out to visit on those evenings. Indeed, their house had an odd look to it: The shades were always drawn and the lawn was seldom mowed. It wasn't that the house was an eyesore, it just wasn't as well cared for as the others. The neighborhood kids told my girls stories about the old couple who lived there.

"They're creepy! They really are!" said the ten-year-old twin boys next door. "When we collected old clothes for the school rummage sale, we rang their bell. The man answered, and we could see into the house. It was completely dark except for this one weird candle in the living room!"

"They dress funny, too," added another girl who lived down the block. "Even when it's really hot out, they always bundle up in long sleeves and high collars."

"And they talk funny!" piped up another little one.

I didn't take any of this talk seriously, and, like the other mothers in the neighborhood, I cautioned my girls about being unkind or rude. When I overheard one of the children jumping rope to a rhyme that made fun of the old woman—"Mrs. Feldman, teeth of yellow, went downtown to meet a fellow"—I put a stop to it. Having eccentrics even made the neighborhood kind of interesting. Not that they included themselves among the neighbors.

One evening toward the end of summer, when the days were beginning to shorten, the girls and I stepped outside after supper to visit with our new friends and breathe the last lingering smells of summer. We were so relaxed and happy that we were completely unprepared for what happened next.

As Rachael opened the gate to the backyard, Lady joined us, barking and circling joyfully in her newfound freedom. But for some reason, instead of basking in the attention of the gathering children, she made a beeline for the one house on the block that would not welcome her. Ignoring our commands, she charged across the street, up the front walk, and right to the front door of the strange old couple.

I dashed after Lady, but stopped suddenly when Mrs. Feldman appeared at the door, brandishing a broom at our dog, screaming something. For a moment, I stood rooted where I was, appalled and terrified. Lady backed away from the hysterical woman, came back to me and sat at my feet. I grabbed her collar.

What should I do? Take my dog straight home? Apologize to our new neighbor, who now stood at the top of her steps shaking all over, tears streaming down her face?

In another second, my husband and children were beside me and Mr. Feldman had appeared, putting an arm around his wife, and ushering her back into the house. The door closed with a thud.

"What was it she screamed?" asked my frightened Rachael. "Is she going to call the police? Are we going to lose Lady?"

I looked down at my daughter's tear-stained face. For a moment, I couldn't answer. Something was becoming clear, but it took a moment to understand what it was.

My parents had spoken Yiddish in my house when I was a little girl. The words Mrs. Feldman had yelled weren't Yiddish, but they were close enough for me to understand. In clear German, she had screamed, "Never again, never again, not the dog!"

That night, I assured the girls we wouldn't lose Lady for such a minor offense. The next day, there seemed a more pressing issue.

"Girls," I said, "we're going over to the Feldmans' house to apologize."

"What if they won't listen?" asked Anna fearfully.

"At least they will hear," I said.

Hand in hand, the three of us climbed the front steps to the Feldmans' house. Rachael rang the bell. When Mr. Feldman opened the door, I immediately wished I had thought to bring something . . . a cake, perhaps. I was afraid he would close the door when he saw who it was.

He didn't.

"We came to apologize to you and your wife for allowing our dog to frighten her so. She got out by accident. We'll make sure it doesn't happen again."

Behind the old man, the house was indeed dark, as the neighborhood children had said; the little candle they'd described was burning in the living room. But I also glimpsed something else. Above the candle, in a little silver picture frame, was an old photo of a little girl.

Mr. Feldman didn't say anything as we finished speaking. From behind him, his wife emerged from the shadow. She looked down at my girls—and smiled.

As we walked home, I knew what I had to explain to my children. We sat down at the kitchen table and talked about the Holocaust. I told them I thought our neighbors were survivors of that terrible time. It explained their reticence, the clothes that they wore, probably covering numbers tattooed into them, their foreign accent. I told them that the candle that burned in the living room was a Jewish memorial candle; we talked about the photo of the little girl.

Something happened to the children after that—not just to my children, but to the whole neighborhood. Word got around. The twins next door began taking turns mowing the Feldmans' lawn. Their newspapers and mail were never left by the street anymore, but placed carefully between their screen and front doors. A pot of geraniums was left on their front porch . . . and Mrs. Feldman began coming outside to water them. Children on bicycles riding past waved at her, and she waved back.

The weather turned cooler, and the leaves began to fall. The children started school. One evening, our family went out together to take Lady for a walk. We had just stepped onto our sidewalk when we saw that Mr. and Mrs. Feldman were leaving their house, too.

Lady barked at them, and just for a minute, I saw them freeze. But in another minute, our neighbors smiled, waved and walked on. For they truly were our neighbors now. Whether we all realized it or not, an exchange had taken place among us, one that was much more important than cakes or flour or even a wave and a smile. For the Feldmans had given our neighborhood a past—and we, in turn, had helped them find a future.

Marsha Arons

Letters to Anne Frank's Father

To keep a lamp burning we have to keep putting oil in it.

Mother Teresa

I sat on my suitcase as the Swiss train carried me to a meeting I'd dreamed of for two decades. At the end of the journey waited Anne Frank's father, Otto, with whom I had corresponded since I was fourteen.

I wanted this encounter with the man I'd come to think of as a second father to be all emotion, embraces, tears. But I realized Otto would probably just shake my hand formally, and we would have a very civilized time together, and that would be that. I was prepared.

The dream of this day had begun to take shape when I was twelve, growing up in California's San Fernando Valley. I had auditioned for the starring role in the 1959 movie *The Diary of Anne Frank*. I didn't get the part, but I found a whole new world in Anne Frank's diary.

Despite the monumental differences in our situations, I identified strongly with this eloquent girl my own age. Her predicament burned in my thoughts: how she hid from the Nazis in a tiny annex above her father's Amsterdam office building, bursting with frustrated life, "like a canary in a cage." How she remained hidden for two years with her parents, Otto and Edith, her older sister, the Van Daan family and a dentist. How they were caught and imprisoned in a concentration camp, where she died. How she still believed, after all she'd been through, that "people are really good at heart."

Two years after first reading her diary, I wrote Otto Frank in Birsfelden, Switzerland, where he and his second wife, Fritzi, eventually settled. Would he answer me? Did he speak English? Could I even talk to him of Anne, or would it be too painful?

Then came a letter. I must have read it a hundred times.

> *August 21, 1959*
>
> *I received your kind letter and thank you for it. Anne's ardent wish was to work for mankind, and therefore an Anne Frank Foundation has been incorporated in Amsterdam to work in her spirit. You are right that I receive many letters from young people all over the world, but you will understand that it is not possible for me to carry on correspondence, though, as you see, I am answering everyone.*
>
> *Wishing you all the best, I am with kindest regards.*
>
> *Yours,*
> *Otto Frank*

I replied that he didn't have to answer me. I would simply write to him whether he answered or not. After that, whenever an attack of "I-can't-take-this-any-longer" hit me, I'd put it all into a lengthy letter. And he always answered.

At fifteen I wrote to him about my wish to be an actress. He replied:

> *Continue to study dancing, continue to work on literature and drama, but let it be your hobby. . . . To have acting and dancing as a job is very difficult.*

In college, where I changed majors as fast as I changed socks, Otto Frank was there for me. From dance to drama to English, my dear distant "guidance counselor" was much more tolerant than those at U.C.L.A.

He was there, too, when I contemplated marrying a man who wasn't Jewish. He advised me to get books about Judaism for my fiancé to read. We did this.

When we married, Otto wrote:

> *Do not mind the disapproval of others. The main thing is that your personalities are well matched and you have respect for each other's conviction.*

Though I was joyous in my marriage, that was the difficult year of 1968. After Robert Kennedy was killed, I wrote:

> *Bobby Kennedy is dead. Martin Luther King, Jr. is dead. John F. Kennedy is dead. Medgar Evers is dead. All shot by madmen. How can I bring a child into this world?*

He wrote back:

> *Never give up! I once read, "If the end of the world were imminent, I still would plant a tree today." Life goes on, and perhaps your child will bring the world one step further.*

In honor of my birthday that year, Mr. Frank sent me a note:

> *Two trees in Israel in the name of Mrs. Cara Wilson for her birthday. Planted by Mr. O. Frank, Birsfelden.*

Otto Frank's vision of hope gave my husband and me the courage to become parents. We had two sons, Ethan and Jesse. My trip to Switzerland was the first time I had been away from them.

The train was slowing. The conductor announced the stop and the doors flew open.

I looked into the crowd and saw a man with a straight back and Lincolnesque face. Snow-white hair surrounded a balding head. A tall, elderly man, still strong and handsome.

It was really him. Otto Frank.

"Cara! At last!" he said warmly. I was actually hugging him. A real bear hug. Thank God. No formal handshakes or polite hellos. Suddenly a little shy, he put his arm in mine. Fritzi linked my other arm, and we walked off.

When I stepped into the Franks' house, I felt that I was home. Otto took me into their little study. A pile of fresh mail lay stacked on his desk. He showed me wall-to-wall notebooks bursting with letters.

Then Otto brought out another notebook. "These are your letters, Cara. I saved them all." I couldn't believe it. I was facing myself through twenty years of letters. I saw my twelve-year-old's scrawl evolve into an adult's script and then change to typewritten pages. Masses of exclamation points and underlinings, outpourings of feeling.

Then Otto said, "You are not the only one to write all these years."

Smiling, he told me about some of the others. There was Sumi from Japan, who had lost her father. She read Anne's diary and was moved to write to Otto. She told him that she would like to become his "letter daughter"—and signed all her letters "Your daughter, Sumi." Otto advised her through the years.

Then there was John Neiman, who, as a college student, reread *Anne Frank: The Diary of a Young Girl* and wrote to

Mr. Frank. Otto told him, "If you want to honor Anne's memory and the people that died, do what Anne wanted so very much—do good for other people."

For John, that meant becoming a priest. Today Father John, a Catholic priest in Redondo Beach, California, continues to reach out to Holocaust survivors.

And there was Vassa. Some time ago Otto had received a letter from Athens. He went to the Greek embassy, where he was referred to a local teacher who translated the letter from Greek.

The young writer told Otto about her horrifying background—how her father, who had been in the underground movement against the Nazis, had been murdered in front of her. Vassa lost interest in everything—in life itself.

Then she saw the play, *The Diary of Anne Frank.* She wrote to Otto, pouring out her heart. He responded that though Anne was deprived of seeing her goals achieved, Vassa had a whole lifetime of promise before her. The correspondence continued, and with Otto's encouragement, Vassa overcame her depression.

Realizing the girl no longer needed his advice, Otto wrote to her explaining the strain it was to have her letters translated. He was getting too old. He had to stop writing her.

For over a year Otto didn't hear from Vassa. Then a letter came, bearing her familiar signature. The letter was in French—a language Otto could read. During those months, Vassa had studied French so she could write to her dear mentor.

Throughout my visit I listened carefully to what Otto said, sensing it would be important to remember everything about this time. As if reading my mind, he told me quietly, "It was good that you came now. I'm an old man, you know."

We continued to correspond for two more years. Then one day I received a letter from Fritzi that began:

> *Dearest Cara,*
>   *Now my darling Otto has left me and all his friends . . .*

I could only marvel at how many lives this gentle man had affected—and feel fortunate that mine had been one of them. We are from different races and religions, but in one way we are the same. After all, were we not sent by Anne to keep her father company?

Cara Wilson

A Reason to Live

In October 1986, farmer Darrell Adams needed help with the corn harvest. He asked his wife, Marilyn, if eleven-year-old Keith, Marilyn's son and Darrell's stepson, could stay home from school to help. Darrell's request wasn't an unusual one in farm country, where children are often needed to help bring in the crops.

Marilyn stifled a sense of foreboding and gave her permission. *Staying home from school to help with the harvest is a rite of passage for a farm kid,* she told herself. Keith had shown his mother he knew the rules of working safely around farm machinery, and the boy was proud that Darrell had asked for his help.

Before she left for a computer class in Des Moines the next morning, Marilyn fixed a big farm breakfast for Keith and Darrell. As she walked out the door she told them, "You guys be careful today. I don't know what I'd do without either one of you."

Later that afternoon, when Darrell rolled his combine into the farmyard to unload more corn, he found Keith curled in the fetal position at the bottom of the grain wagon, 14,000 pounds of corn on top of him and kernels clogging his throat. In a panic, Darrell rushed Keith to the nearby medical clinic, where medics did what they could for the boy while a hospital helicopter flew to the rescue.

Marilyn had been rousted from her computer class to take the telephone call all parents fear. She was driven to the hospital, dread cloaking her like a shroud. Darrell, who had been driven to the hospital by clinic personnel, met her there.

"I killed him! I killed him!" he cried, as he buried his face in his big, rough farmers' hands.

At Keith's bedside, Marilyn anxiously examined her son, his eighty-pound body shaking from shock, his face almost covered by the oxygen mask. Keith was hooked up to every medical device imaginable and an intravenous bag hung from a metal stand over his head. As Marilyn brushed her son's hair from his forehead, she noticed that his face felt cold and clammy. She felt his arms, legs and feet—they were like ice.

Stricken and helpless, Marilyn sat and prayed for Keith, who had read the Bible cover to cover and wanted to be a minister. Several hours into her vigil, she leaned over and spoke to her son.

"Keith," she said. "We have to talk to Jesus now."

A single tear fell from the corner of the boy's left eye and ran down his cheek.

At 2:30 A.M., with Marilyn on one side of his bed and his grandmother on the other, Keith stopped trembling. Marilyn felt her precious boy slip away to a place beyond pain and suffering. Her only son was gone.

Marilyn sank into sorrow so deep that even her family's love and concern could not reach her. She stopped going to church because all she did was cry. She couldn't drag herself to school programs or go to parent-teacher conferences. Her remaining daughters had to parent her. She watched, numb with grief, as she and Darrell grew apart.

It was a request for help from her daughter, Kelly, that started Marilyn on her road to recovery. Kelly had joined FFA, Future Farmers of America, which teaches young people about agriculture and related occupations. Her younger brother's death had spurred Kelly to do a presentation on the dangers of grain wagons.

Together, mother and daughter researched the subject and found a recommendation that warning decals should be placed on the side of grain wagons. No one, they found to their surprise and consternation, had followed up on the recommendation. No one, that is, until Marilyn Adams decided that she and her family would do it.

Marilyn realized she could resurrect her son's memory, if not his life, by spreading the word about the dangers of farming for children. A woman with a mission, Marilyn channeled her profound sense of loss into starting an organization called Farm Safety 4 Just Kids.

Her employer donated enough money to print the warning decals Marilyn and her family had designed, sitting around their kitchen table. Iowa FFA chapters distributed thousands of these decals, sticking them on grain wagons while farmers waited in line to unload at grain elevators across Iowa. Marilyn felt reborn. She had found a reason to live and a way to keep Keith's memory alive.

Marilyn knew that there was still a lot of hard work ahead. Garnering the support of the Iowa Farm Safety Council, she did a radio interview, and then a couple of articles appeared in farm magazines on Marilyn and her fledgling organization. The publicity prompted a flood of phone calls from the public and the media.

"The phone just rang and rang and rang. We couldn't even eat dinner. A lot of people called who'd lost a child in a farming accident. They wanted to talk to me and reach out. Many of the people who get involved in Farm Safety 4 Just Kids have also lost children in farm

accidents—it helps them in their grief. Any time a griev-
ing parent calls me, I put them to work. It gives us something positive to do in our lives. That was when I began to
feel I had a purpose in life, like I could begin to nurture
again," Marilyn recalls.

Marilyn tirelessly traveled the country, talking to busi-
nesses. She eventually lined up enough financial support
so she could quit her job and work on farm safety issues
full-time. She convinced then-First Lady Barbara Bush to
be honorary chairwoman of Farm Safety 4 Just Kids.

"Nobody says 'no' to Marilyn Adams," Mrs. Bush said.

Over the last ten years, the organization has grown
enormously. Today Farm Safety 4 Just Kids has a staff of
nine, an annual budget of $750,000 and seventy-seven
chapters in the United States and Canada.

And recently, a study found that farm accidents
claimed the lives of 39 percent fewer children since the
founding of Farm Safety 4 Just Kids. There are many reasons for the decline, but most of the experts agree that
Farm Safety 4 Just Kids is one of them.

Fulfilled with her success, her family whole and happy
once more—Marilyn and Darrell even had another baby—
Marilyn seems at peace. When asked how she envisioned
Keith in heaven, Marilyn laughed and said, "I believe he's
very busy pointing his mother in the right direction."

Jerry Perkins

[EDITORS' NOTE: *For more information about Farm Safety*
4 Just Kids, write to P.O. Box 458, Earlham, IA 50072 or call
515-758-2827.]

The Night I Wrote
My Pulitzer Prize Winner

*I long to accomplish a great and noble task, but
it is my chief duty to accomplish small tasks as
if they were great and noble.*

Helen Keller

As a writer, I've felt that someday, somewhere my work
would touch human hearts, bridge continents, unite generations. One night, it did.

I'm at McKelvey's Tavern, sipping Amber Bock. The
Blues Band is on a break. A small, white-haired man sits
two barstools away.

"I've got ten kids," he boasts. "And two grandbabies on
the way. My youngest daughter is in the Army. I think the
world of that girl. Last five years, she's been in Germany."

"Does she call you?"

"Sometimes. But with her schedule and the time difference, we don't talk much anymore." His lips tighten as he
looks into his beer. "It costs a bundle to phone over there.
She tells me, 'Call collect, Dad.' Nah, I can't put that
expense on her."

"Write a letter," I suggest.

"Can't hold a pen," he says. "I've had four strokes. My arm is paralyzed." To show me, he lifts the lifeless limb with his good hand.

I grab my journal, open to a clean page, and lean forward, pen in hand. "What's her name?"

"Suzie."

I look into his bloodshot eyes and ask, "Shall I start with 'Dear Suzie,' 'Hi Suzie,' or 'Suzie, how the heck are ya?'?"

"All of that." He grins, exhales smoke.

"Dear Suzie," I slowly repeat, then pen the words. "You talk, I'll write."

He presses the bit stub of his cigarette into the small tin ashtray, reaches for another Camel, lights up and inhales. "Tell her I'm down to one pack a day ... and ... I eat every day . . . at the Senior Center. The food is wonderful. Spaghetti, cake, ice cream. All you can eat." He adds with a chuckle, "Just no beer."

I listen and write nonstop.

"Tell her I think the world of her. Tell her Jen and Dave are getting married and Pat and Tim are getting divorced. Tell her Uncle Wilbur is still up on Doe Island, workin' the pumpkin patch. That's where all my kids grew up."

As I listen, a kind of intimacy opens between the wizened-faced man and me.

"Tell her not to worry. I've got no complaints. I dance every night I can." His eyes sparkle. "Tell her to remember Grandpa Jones. He died jogging—at 104. That gives me more than twenty years. Tell her . . . I think the world of her." His voice quivers. He gulps his beer, wipes his mouth.

Two blank lines remain on the second side of the paper. I pick up his limp arm, place my pen in his rigid hand, and squeeze his fingers. "You sign it," I urge.

To add leverage, he couches his left hand around his writing hand. I watch him etch each stroke. The scribble reads "Jove Da." I know he means "Love, Dad." The pen rolls out of his hand. His right arm flops to his side. With his left arm, he reaches a finger beneath his glasses, wipes a tear.

"Thanks," he says in a half-whisper, then clears his throat.

"No big deal. I write in this journal every day." I pat his shoulder and leave, saying, "When the Blues Band plays next Saturday, you bring Suzie's address. I'll bring a stamped envelope."

On the way home, I wept. I knew I had just written my Pulitzer Prize winner.

Shinan Barclay

A Perfect Pot of Tea

There are high spots in all of our lives and most of them have come about through encouragement from someone else. I don't care how great, how famous or successful a man or woman may be, each hungers for applause.

George M. Adams

An impatient crowd of nearly 200 diehard bargain hunters shoved their way into the huge living room of the old Withers homestead. The sweltering ninety-degree temperature didn't deter a single one, all in pursuit of the estate-sale find of the summer.

The lady conducting the sale, a long-time acquaintance, nodded as we watched the early-morning scavengers. "How's this for bedlam?" she chuckled.

I smiled in agreement. "I shouldn't even be here. I have to be at the airport in less than an hour," I admitted to her. "But when I was a teenager, I sold cosmetics in this neighborhood. And Hillary Withers was my favorite customer."

"Then run and check out the attic," she suggested. "There are plenty of old cosmetics up there."

Quickly, I squeezed through the ever-growing throng and climbed the stairs to the third floor. The attic was deserted except for a petite, elderly woman presiding over several tables loaded with yellowed bags of all sizes.

"What brings you all the way up here?" she asked, as she popped the stopper out of a perfume bottle. "There's nothing up here except old Avon, Tupperware and Fuller Brush products."

I drew in a long, cautious breath. The unmistakable fragrance of "Here's My Heart" perfume transported me back nearly twenty years.

"Why, this is my own handwriting!" I exclaimed, as my eyes fell upon an invoice stapled to one of the bags. The untouched sack held more than a hundred dollars' worth of creams and colognes—my very first sale to Mrs. Withers.

On that long-ago June day, I'd canvassed the wide, tree-lined avenue for nearly four hours, but not one lady of the house had invited me indoors. Instead, several had slammed their doors in my face. As I rang the bell at the last house, I braced myself for the now-familiar rejection.

"Hello, ma'am, I'm your new Avon representative," I stammered, when the carved-oak door swung open. "I have some great products I'd like to show you." When my eyes finally found the courage to face the lady in the doorway, I realized it was Mrs. Withers, the bubbly, matronly soprano in our church choir. I'd admired her lovely dresses and hats, dreaming that someday I'd wear stylish clothes, too.

Just two months before, when I'd traveled to a distant city to have brain surgery, Mrs. Withers had showered me with the most beautiful cards. Once she'd even tucked in a Scripture verse: "I can do all things through Christ which strengtheneth me." I'd carried it in my red vinyl wallet. Whenever my teachers told me I'd never make it to college, I'd take it out and study it, repeating its promise softly to myself.

I'd believed that verse, even when my teachers kept saying, "With all the school you've missed, Roberta, you can never catch up." Perhaps they felt it was kinder not to let me dream too much, because I was afflicted with neurofibromatosis, a serious neurological disorder.

"Why, Roberta dear, come in, come in," Mrs. Withers's voice sang out. "I need a million and one things. I'm so glad you came to see me."

Gingerly, I eased myself onto the spotless white sofa and unzipped my tweed satchel filled with all the cosmetics samples five dollars could buy. When I handed Mrs. Withers a sales brochure, suddenly I felt like the most important girl in the world.

"Mrs. Withers, we have two types of creams, one for ruddy skin tones and another for sallow skin," I explained with newfound confidence. "And they're great for wrinkles, too."

"Oh good, good," she chanted.

"Which one would you like to try?" I asked as I started to adjust the wig hiding my stubbly, surgery-scarred scalp.

"Oh, I'll surely need one of each," she answered. "And what do you have in the way of fragrances?"

"Here, try this one, Mrs. Withers. They recommend that you place it on the pulse point for the best effect," I instructed, pointing to her diamond-and-gold-clad wrist.

"Why, Roberta, you're so knowledgeable about all of this. You must have studied for days. What an intelligent young woman you are."

"You really think so, Mrs. Withers?"

"Oh, I know so. And just what do you plan to do with your earnings?"

"I'm saving for college to be a registered nurse," I replied, surprised at my own words. "But today, I'm thinking more of buying my mother a cardigan sweater for her birthday. She always goes with me for my medical treatments, and when we travel on the train, a sweater would be nice for her."

"Wonderful, Roberta, and so considerate. Now what do you have in the gifts line?" she asked, requesting two of each item I recommended.

Her extravagant order totaled $117.42. Had she meant to order so much? I wondered. But she smiled and said, "I'll look forward to receiving my delivery, Roberta. Did you say next Tuesday?"

I was preparing to leave when Mrs. Withers said, "You look absolutely famished. Would you like some tea before you go? At our house, we think of tea as liquid sunshine."

I nodded, then followed Mrs. Withers to her pristine kitchen, filled with all manner of curiosities. I watched, spellbound, as she orchestrated a tea party, like those I'd seen in the movies, just for me. She carefully filled the tea kettle with cold water, brought it to a "true" boil, then let the tea leaves steep for "exactly" five long minutes. "So the flavor will blossom," she explained.

Then she arranged a silver tray with a delicate china tea set, a chintz tea cozy, tempting strawberry scones and other small splendors. At home, we sometimes drank iced tea in jelly glasses, but never had I felt like a princess invited to afternoon tea.

"Excuse me, Mrs. Withers, but isn't there a faster way to fix tea?" I asked. "At home, we use tea bags."

Mrs. Withers wrapped her arm around my shoulders. "There are some things in life that shouldn't be hurried," she confided. "I've learned that brewing a proper pot of tea is a lot like living a life that pleases God. It takes extra effort, but it's always worth it.

"Take you, for instance, with all of your health problems. Why, you're steeped with determination and ambition, just like a perfect pot of tea. Many in your shoes would give up, but not you. And with God's help, you can accomplish anything you set your mind to, Roberta."

Abruptly, my journey back in time ended when the lady in the hot, sticky attic asked, "You knew Hillary Withers, too?"

I wiped a stream of perspiration from my forehead. "Yes . . . I once sold her some of these cosmetics. But I can't understand why she never used them or gave them away."

"She did give a lot of them away," the lady replied matter-of-factly, "but somehow, some of them got missed and ended up here."

"But why did she buy them and not use them?" I asked.

"Oh, she purchased a special brand of cosmetics for her own use." The lady spoke in a confidential whisper. "Hillary had a soft spot in her heart for door-to-door salespeople. She never turned any of them away. She used to tell me, 'I could just give them money, but money alone doesn't buy self-respect. So I give them a little of my money, lend a listening ear, and share my love and prayers. You never know how far a little encouragement can take someone.'"

I paused, remembering how my cosmetics sales had soared after I'd first visited Mrs. Withers. I bought my mother the new sweater from my commission on the sale, and I still had enough money for my college fund. I even went on to win several district and national cosmetics-sales awards. Eventually, I put myself through college with my own earnings and realized my dream of becoming a registered nurse. Later, I earned a master's degree and a Ph.D.

"Mrs. Withers prayed for all of these people?" I asked, pointing to the dozens of time-worn delivery bags on the table.

"Oh, yes," she assured me. "She did it without the slightest yearning that anyone would ever know."

I paid the cashier for my purchases—the sack of cosmetics I'd sold to Mrs. Withers, and a tiny, heart-shaped gold locket. I threaded the locket onto the gold chain I wore around my neck. Then I headed for the airport; later that afternoon, I was addressing a medical convention in New York.

When I arrived in the elegant hotel ballroom, I found my way to the speaker's podium and scanned the sea of faces—health care specialists from all over the country. Suddenly, I felt as insecure as on that long-ago day, peddling cosmetics in that unfamiliar, affluent neighborhood.

Can I do it? my mind questioned.

My trembling fingers reached upward to the locket. It opened, revealing a picture of Mrs. Withers inside. I again heard her soft but emphatic words: "With God's help, you can accomplish anything you set your mind to, Roberta."

"Good afternoon," I began slowly. "Thank you for inviting me to speak about putting the care back in health care. It's often said that nursing is love made visible. But this morning I learned an unexpected lesson about the power of quiet love expressed in secret. The kind of love expressed not for show, but for the good it can do in the lives of others. Some of our most important acts of love, sometimes, go unnoticed. Until they've had time to steep—for their flavor to blossom."

Then I told my colleagues the story of Hillary Withers. To my surprise, there was thunderous applause. Silently, I prayed, *Thank you, God, and Mrs. Withers.* And to think it all began with a perfect pot of tea.

Roberta Messner, R.N., Ph.D.

7

OVERCOMING OBSTACLES

Walk on a rainbow trail; walk on a trail of song, and all about you will be beauty. There is a way out of every dark mist, over a rainbow trail.

Navajo Song

Lunch with Helen Keller

My husband and I loved our house in Italy. It sat high on a cliff above Portofino with an extraordinary view of the blue harbor below, and its white beach was surrounded by cypresses. There was, however, a serpent in our paradise: the path up the cliff. The municipal authorities refused to grant us permission to build a proper road in lieu of the mule track. The only vehicle that could climb the narrow path and negotiate the hairpin turns, the steep incline and the potholes, was an old American Army jeep we had bought in Genoa. It possessed neither springs nor brakes. When you wanted to stop, you had to go into reverse and back up against something. But it was indestructible, and you could rely on it in all weathers.

One day in the summer of 1950, our neighbor, Contessa Margot Besozzi, who of necessity also owned a jeep, called to say that her cousin had arrived in town with a companion and that her own jeep had conked out. Would I mind going to fetch the two old ladies in ours? They were at the Hotel Splendido.

"Whom should I ask for at the hotel?" I asked.

"Miss Helen Keller."

"Who?"

"Miss Helen Keller, K-e-l-l . . . "

"Margot, you don't mean *Helen Keller?*"

"Of course," she said. "She's my cousin. Didn't you know?"

I ran into the garage, jumped into the jeep and raced down the mountain.

I had been twelve years old when my father gave me the book about Helen Keller written by Anne Sullivan, the remarkable woman whom fate had chosen to be the teacher of the blind and deaf child. Anne Sullivan had turned the rebellious, brutish little child into a civilized member of society by teaching her to speak. I still remembered vividly her description of the first few months of physical battle with the child, until the glorious moment when she held Helen's left hand under a running water tap and the blind, deaf and up until then mute little girl made history by stammering out an intelligible word: "Wa-ter."

Over the years I had read about Helen Keller in the newspapers. I knew that Anne Sullivan was no longer with her and that a new companion now accompanied her everywhere. But the few minutes it took me to drive down the hill were not nearly enough to get used to the idea that I was going to meet in person this mythical figure from my early youth.

I backed the jeep up against a bougainvillaea-covered wall and presented myself at the hotel. A tall, buxom, vigorous-looking woman rose from a chair on the hotel terrace to greet me: Polly Thomson, Helen Keller's companion. A second figure rose slowly from the chair beside her and held out her hand. Helen Keller, then in her seventies, was a slight, white-haired woman with wide-open blue eyes and a shy smile.

"How do you do?" she said slowly and a little gutturally.

I took her hand, which she was holding too high because she didn't know how tall I was. She was bound to make this mistake with people she was meeting for the first time, but she never made it twice. Later, when we said good-bye, she put her hand firmly into mine at exactly the right level.

The luggage was loaded into the back of the jeep, and I helped the jolly Miss Thomson to sit beside it. The hotel porter lifted Helen Keller's fragile body and set it down on the front seat next to me. Only then did it dawn on me that this was going to be a risky undertaking. The jeep was open; there was nothing you could hold onto properly. How was I to keep the blind and deaf woman from falling out of the rickety old thing when we took a curve, which had to be done at a fast clip because of the angle and the jeep's general condition? I turned to her and said, "Miss Keller, I must prepare you—we're going up a very steep hill. Can you hold tight to this piece of metal on the windshield?"

But she continued to look expectantly straight ahead. Behind me, Miss Thomson said patiently, "She can't hear you, dear, nor see you. I know it's hard to get used to it at first."

I was so embarrassed that I stammered like an idiot, trying to explain the problem ahead of us. All the while, Miss Keller never turned her head or seemed puzzled by the delay. She sat motionless, a slight smile on her face, patiently waiting. Miss Thomson knelt across the luggage and reached for her hand. Rapidly she moved Helen's fingers up, down and sideways, telling her in blind-deaf language what I had just said.

"I don't mind," said Helen, laughing. "I'll hold tight."

I took courage, got hold of her hands, and placed them on the piece of metal in front of her. "Okay," she cried gaily, and I switched on the ignition. The jeep started with a jump and Miss Thomson fell off her seat on top of the luggage. I couldn't stop and help her up because of the steep hill, the dangerous curve ahead and the absence of brakes. We roared upward, my eyes glued to the narrow path, and Miss Thomson helpless as a beetle on its back.

I'd had plenty of passengers in the jeep, and they'd all complained about the lack of springs. No wonder, with all those boulders and potholes, not to mention the hairpin turns through the olive trees, which only partially obscured the precipitous drop that had unnerved quite a few of our guests. Helen was the first passenger who was oblivious to the danger; she was enchanted by the violent jumps and only laughed when she was thrown against my shoulder. Helen actually began to sing. "This is fun," she warbled happily, bouncing up and down. "Lovely!" she cried.

We tore past our house at breakneck speed—out of the corner of my eye I saw our gardener, Giuseppe, crossing himself—and continued onward and upward. I had no idea how Miss Thomson was doing, for the jeep's fearful roar had long ago drowned out her anguished protests. But I knew that Helen was still next to me. Her thin white hair had come undone and fluttered about her face, and she was enjoying the crazy ride like a child riding up and down on a wooden horse on a merry-go-round.

At last we rounded the last curve between two giant fig trees, and I could see Margot and her husband waiting for us at their entrance gate. Helen was lifted out of the jeep and hugged; the luggage was unloaded, and Miss Thomson upended and dusted off.

I was invited to lunch. While the two old ladies were being shown to their rooms to freshen up, Margot told me about her cousin and her life. Helen was famous the world over, and in every civilized country, the great and the renowned were eager to meet her and do something for her. Heads of state, scholars and artists vied to receive her, and she had traveled all over the world to satisfy her burning curiosity.

"But don't forget," said Margot, "all she really notices is a change of smell. Whether she's here or in New York or in India, she sits in a black, silent hole."

Arm in arm, casually, as if they just happened to be fond of each other, the two old ladies walked through the garden toward the terrace, where we were waiting for them.

"That must be wisteria," said Helen, "and masses of it, too. I recognize the scent."

I went to pick a large bunch of the blossoms, which surrounded the terrace, and laid it in her lap. "I knew it!" she cried happily, touching them.

Of course, Helen's diction was not quite normal. She spoke haltingly, like someone who has had a stroke, and her consonants were slow and labored. She turned to me, looking directly at me because she had sensed where I was sitting. "You know, we're on the way to Florence to see Michelangelo's David. I'm so thrilled; I've always wanted to see it."

Mystified, I looked at Miss Thomson, who nodded.

"It's true," she said. "The Italian government has had a scaffolding erected around the statue so that Helen can climb up and touch it. That's what she calls 'seeing.' We often go to the theater in New York, and I tell her what's going on onstage and describe the actors. Sometimes we go backstage, too, so that she can 'see' the sets and the actors. Then she goes home, feeling that she's really witnessed the performance."

All the time we were talking, Helen sat and waited. Now and then, when our conversation went on too long, I saw her thin fingers take her friend's hand inquiringly, never impatiently.

Luncheon was served on the terrace. Helen was led to her chair, and I watched her "see" her place setting. Quick as lightning, her hands moved over the objects on the table—plate, glass, silverware—memorizing where they were. Never once during the meal did she grope about; she reached out casually and firmly like the rest of us.

After lunch, we stayed on the shady terrace, surrounded by trailing clusters of wisteria like a thick mauve curtain, the sun below us glittering on the sea. Helen sat in the usual way, head raised slightly as though listening to something, her sightless blue eyes wide open. Her face, although an old lady's face, had something of a schoolgirl's innocence. Whatever suffering must have tormented her—and might still torment her, for all I knew— her face showed no trace of it. It was an isolated face, a saintly face.

I asked her, through her friend, what else she wanted to see in Italy. Then she slowly mapped out her Italian journey—all the places she wanted to visit and the people she would meet. Incredibly, she spoke French quite well and could make herself understood in German and Italian. Sculpture was, naturally, her favorite form of art, because she could touch it and experience it firsthand.

"There's still so much I'd like to see," she said, "so much to learn. And death is just around the corner. Not that that worries me. On the contrary."

"Do you believe in life after death?" I asked.

"Most certainly," she said emphatically. "It is no more than passing from one room into another."

We sat in silence.

Suddenly, Helen spoke again. Slowly and very distinctly she said, "But there's a difference for me, you know. Because in that other room, I shall be able to see."

Lilli Palmer

One Kid at a Time

*Patience and perseverance have a magical effect
before which difficulties disappear and obstacles
vanish.*

John Quincy Adams

I consider myself a simple person. I love my husband
and my children, and I positively dote on my grandchildren. I just have a soft spot for kids—all kids.
Especially kids who are born with physical problems.
They can't help their situation, and it seems to me that
they deserve to enjoy life as much as anyone.

My nephew, Stevie, was born without sweat glands, a
condition called HED. That meant that any exertion could
cause his body to overheat and seriously damage his system. Playing could actually kill him! It was a horrible task
to keep a young child from "overdoing it." He couldn't
understand why we wouldn't let him have fun and run
around like the other children. What kid can live without
playing?

Distraught, one day I wailed to my husband, "If we can
put a man on the moon, there must be *something* we can

do for Stevie!" That set me thinking, and the logical con-clusion of *that* chain of thought was NASA. "I'm going to call NASA," I said firmly.

My startled husband scoffed, *"You're* going to call NASA? Honey, you're a housewife. What are you going to say to NASA?"

I didn't know exactly, but I figured it was worth a try. So I called them. It was amazing, but somehow, I got through to someone who could help me. When I explained Stevie's problem, the man on the other end of the line considered for a moment and then told me about the "cool suit." They'd used it on a few of the moon mis-sions, and he thought it might do the trick for Stevie. I was thrilled.

But there's always a catch—the cool suit cost $2,600. Twenty-six hundred dollars we certainly did not have. But I knew I'd just have to find the money. I had to.

So I did. I had bake sales and garage sales and sold hot dogs and hamburgers outside the local Sam's Club. Slowly, the money began to pile up. We bought the cool suit and fitted our little man in it. He was eight years old then and the look on his face when we told him he could help his dad with the lawn work was worth everything. Next he took off on his bicycle and flew down the side-walk on wings of joy.

NASA followed Stevie's progress with interest. They were thrilled with the opportunity to use space tech-nology in this way. They asked if they could put together a documentary about Stevie and the cool suit, and we agreed.

When that documentary aired, I was inundated with letters and calls from parents of children with HED. All asking me to "Please help my child." I couldn't turn my back on all those desperate families. I knew too well the pain they felt.

So I started a foundation in order to raise money for those children to each have their own cool suits. We still raised money the old-fashioned way, but now I could approach corporations as well as individuals. I asked them all, often and urgently, to give what they could to make a child's life "livable" again.

That was over ten years ago. Stevie has grown into a fine young man, getting ready to go to college. He still wears his cool suit when he's going camping or fishing. I tease him that he'd better keep it handy now that he has a girlfriend!

The foundation is still going strong too. So far we've helped over 400 kids with a number of different rare conditions to have more normal lives. Each case is different and requires individual attention. Just last year, I heard about an English family with two little boys, Kyle, six, and Ryan, four, who have a skin condition called XP. The boys could not be exposed to *any* ultraviolet rays, or they ran the risk of almost certain skin cancer. They could never play outside in the sunlight and had to stay indoors in darkened rooms, as even a forty-watt light bulb was considered dangerous for them.

Again, NASA's space technology saved the day. They fitted the boys out in little astronaut suits that completely protected them from UV rays. Then the boys had their first daylight outing—at Disney World! Their smiles were nearly as bright as the gorgeous sunshine they basked in that day.

The people at NASA called me two years ago and asked me if I would be a consultant for them. Me! A housewife and a grandmother—who never went to college. I laughed, but they were serious. One of the men I'd been in contact with there, Mr. Calloway, said I had the mind of an engineer. He told me that the way I approached problems was as effective as any methods he'd observed. He said, "Sarah, if you had been pointed in that direction when you were in school, you would probably be working here at NASA on the space program today. We can always use a good mind here."

I don't know about that, but I do know that when some problem comes up, there's always a part of me that says, "I can do it!" loud and clear. And if I run into problems or get discouraged, I hear an inner voice saying, "Don't you give up yet!" I know that I could never *really* quit—there isn't anyone else championing these kids. Their diseases are too rare or obscure for the regular helping organizations.

It's amazing what can start from a single phone call. Stevie's suffering spurred me to find a way to help. It seems so obvious now, but ten years ago, NASA simply hadn't known that they held the key to let so many children live like children again—able to play and run and smell the sweet air outside.

As a wife and mother, a concerned relative—and now as a NASA consultant—I know that I was put here to do this work: to improve the lives of these children, one kid at a time.

Sarah Ann Reeves Moody

Low-Fat and Happy

They can conquer who believe they can.

Virgil

When you're a kid, it's tough being different. By the time I was ten, I was taller than most kids and overweight. It was then that I began to hide my eating. I felt bad enough about my size, but when the others laughed at me, it only made me feel worse, and I turned to food for comfort.

For a time I tried slumping, so that I'd be closer to my friends' sizes, but my mother wouldn't allow it. Mom always said to me, "Be proud of your height. You've never seen a short model, have you?" *That* got my attention. To me, the word "model" stood for beauty, which certainly wasn't included in the vocabulary I would have used to describe myself.

One day, I was crying about how some of my friends got attention from boys that I didn't. Mom sat me down again. I remember the soft, comforting look in her beautiful baby-blue eyes as she told me the story of *The Ugly*

Duckling—how the little bird's beauty was revealed when its time arrived. Mom told me that we all have our time on earth to shine. "This is their time," she said. "Your time will come when you become a woman." I listened to Mama's story over and over throughout my growing-up years, but my time never really seemed to come.

Grown and married, I started to have my babies. After the birth of each of my three sons, I always hung on to twenty pounds. When I got pregnant with my last son, I went into the pregnancy weighing 209. After that, for a period of eight years, I gave up on ever being a normal weight again. I was the first to crack jokes about my size, laughing with the others on the outside but crying intensely on the inside. I hid my eating binges from my family, hating myself for what I was doing, but unable to control myself.

At the age of thirty-four, I weighed 300 pounds. I was in pain twenty-four hours a day, with degenerative disc problems. My body felt stretched and crushed all at the same time. Stepping on the scales at 300 pounds was a turning point in my life. The scale registered that enormous number, but I felt like a zero. And I realized with startling clarity that if I didn't gain control of my life, I wouldn't be around much longer. I thought of my precious sons—I wouldn't be there to watch them grow up. I'd miss their first crushes, first heartaches, proms, driver's licenses, graduations, weddings—I'd never hold my grandbabies. At that moment, I knew I had two choices: live or die. Something inside me broke free and I heard myself screaming, "I'm going to live! I deserve to live, live, *live!*"

I screamed loud enough to awaken a new me. How I wanted to live that day! I had a drive inside I'd never felt before. I knew then that I was going to do everything in my power to win this battle. I wasn't going to give up on me ever again.

This powerful force inside me for life was a force of love as well. I felt a spark of love for myself—as I was—that had been gone for a long time. I decided, for the first time ever, that I was going to lose weight the healthy way. In the past, I had abused diets as much as I'd abused food. I had starved the weight off to the point of losing my hair and developing blurred vision.

This time, I would set small goals, so that when I reached them it would give me the confidence to continue. I learned to prepare and enjoy low-fat, healthy foods. I also developed a new way to talk to myself about food. When food "called out to me," instead of saying, *Go ahead, girl, eat. Who's going to know?* the new Teresa was firm. *No! I will not eat in private and guilty silence anymore. I will eat when I choose, not when food dictates.* How wonderful it felt when I made it through another day without cheating.

Toughest of all, I had to concentrate on the positives in my life. I had always been so good at encouraging others; now I realized the person who needed me most was me. I made myself wear make-up because it made me feel prouder of myself. Somedays that was just the little push I needed to get me through. As the weight came off and I got smaller, my confidence in myself grew and grew.

I remember the first time I went to the regular, not plus size, section of the local department store. I cried as I looked around at all the racks of clothes I knew I could wear. I grabbed twenty outfits and went to the dressing room. The attendant raised her eyebrows in surprise, saying, "All of these?"

I smiled broadly. "*All* of these," I answered proudly.

Zipping up a pair of jeans, I felt a wonderful sense of freedom. *I'm going to make it,* I thought.

In nine months, I lost 108 pounds, but then I hit a plateau. For years I had blamed my weight on a slow metabolism, and had always fought exercise like I fought losing weight. Now I knew I couldn't go any further without getting my body moving. I remember telling myself, *Girl, you weren't blessed with a great metabolism, but you were blessed with two legs, so get out there and do something about that slow metabolism.* So I did.

Parking my car near a wheat field by my home, I walked along the fence till I reached the end of the one-mile long field. If I wanted to get home, I had to get back to my car, so I had no choice but to walk the return mile. It was hard at first, but it got easier and easier as the weeks and months went by.

Within another eight months, I was at my target weight of 170 pounds. I had lost 130 pounds! At five feet, eleven inches, I am a size twelve. Best of all, I am alive not only in body but in spirit as well.

Now, my husband flirts with me, and our kids think we act weird because we're so happy together. Plus, I'm able to be the active mom with my sons the way I'd always dreamed. We fish, play ball or just hang out together, and amazingly, I have the energy to keep up.

Today, at age thirty-six, I'm blessed with a new career. Writing and publishing my low-fat cookbook has been one of the most exciting adventures I have ever been on. Because of the book and the motivational speaking I do to promote it, I've been given the opportunity to reach out to others who, like I once had, have all but given up hope of losing weight and gaining control of their lives.

For me, losing weight was about choosing life over and over and over again. I remember a day on one of my walks by the wheat field, when I reached over the fence and grabbed a stem of wheat to hold in my hand as I walked. I remembered from school that, to the ancient Greeks, wheat represented life. Whenever I felt like giving up that day, I looked at the wheat in my hand and it spurred me on to finish my two-mile hike.

I still have that piece of wheat. When I have a tough day, I look at it and it reminds me of a girl, and later a woman, who for years thought there was no hope, but through faith, courage and love, found her hope—and her life—again. It is, finally, my time to shine.

Teresa Collins

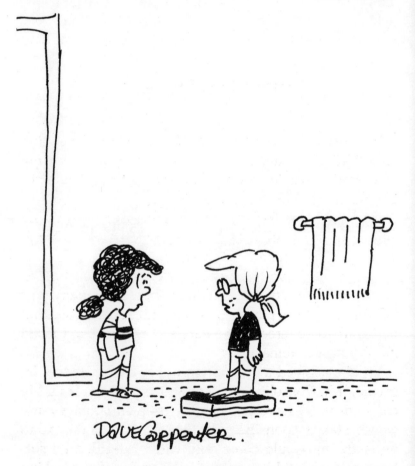

"I think Mom sets the scale back.
I didn't weigh anything until I was five."

Reprinted by permission of Dave Carpenter.

Graduation Message

I'm a divorce lawyer. At times, I feel as if I've heard and seen it all. But ten years ago, a woman walked into my office with a whole new agenda, and neither my life nor my practice has been the same since.

Her name was Barbara, and as she was shown to my office, wearing a rather "plain Jane" outfit, I guessed her to be about nineteen and fairly innocent.

I was wrong. She was thirty-two, with four children between the ages of three and nine. I've heard many brutal stories, but the physical, mental and sexual abuse that Barbara had suffered at the hands of her husband made me sick to my stomach.

Yet she finished a description of her circumstances by saying, "Mr. Concolino, you know, it isn't all his fault. My children and I have remained in this situation by my choice; I take responsibility for that. I've known the end to my suffering would come only when I decided I'd suffered enough, and I've made that decision. I'm breaking the cycle."

I'd been practicing law for fifteen years at that point, and I've got to admit that in my head, I was getting great pleasure from thoughts of nailing that guy to the wall.

"Do you believe in forgiveness, Mr. Concolino?" she asked.

"Yes, of course," I said. "I believe what goes around comes around, and if we try to do the right thing, good comes back to us. The clients of mine who have withheld forgiveness have withheld it only from themselves."

Those words were so common for me that they practically spoke themselves. And yet, if anyone had cause to be full of rage, Barbara did.

"I believe in forgiveness, too," she said quietly. "I believe that if I hold on to anger at my husband, it will only fuel the fire of conflict, and my children are the ones who will get burned."

She gave a tremulous smile. "The problem is, kids are very smart. They can tell if I haven't truly forgiven their dad ... if I am just saying words. So I have to really release my anger.

"And here is where I need a favor from you."

I leaned forward across my desk.

"I don't want this divorce to be bitter. I don't want all the blame put onto him. The thing I most want is to truly forgive him, and to have both you and me conduct ourselves accordingly." She paused and looked me in the eye. "And I want you to promise to hold me to this."

I've got to say, this request was against my best lawyerly business advice. But it fit my best human advice, hand in glove.

"I'll do my best," I said.

It wasn't easy. Barbara's husband had no interest in taking the high road. The next decade was marked with his ugly character assassinations of her and repeated periods of nonpayment of child support. There were even times she could have had him thrown in jail, but she never would.

After yet another court session that went in her favor, she caught me in a corridor. "You've kept your promise, Bob," she said, and she laughed. "I admit that there have been times I've wanted to curse you for making me stick to my beliefs. I still wonder sometimes if it's been worth it. But thanks."

I knew what she meant. In my opinion, her ex continued to violate normal standards of decency. Yet she had never responded in kind.

Barbara ultimately found and married the love of her life. Although matters were settled legally, I always enjoyed getting her Christmas card, hearing how the family was doing.

Then one day I received a call. "Bob, it's Barbara. I need to come in and show you something."

"Of course," I said.

Now what? I thought. *How long is this guy going to keep at this? How long before she finally cracks?*

The woman who walked into my office was lovely and poised, full of so much more confidence than she had possessed ten years earlier. There even seemed to be a bounce to her step.

As I stood to greet her, she handed me a photo—an eight-by-ten taken during her oldest son's senior year in high school. John was wearing his football uniform; his father stood to his left rigidly and coldly. The boy himself was looking proudly at his mom, who stood close to him, a warm smile on her face. I knew from her Christmas letters that he had graduated from a very well-respected private high school.

"This was after he caught the winning touchdown in the championship game," she grinned. "Did I mention that game gave their team the number-one ranking in America?"

"I think I heard something about it," I smiled.

"Read the back," she said.

I turned the photograph over to see what her son had written.

> Mom,
>
> I want you to know that you have been the best mom and dad a boy could ever have. I know because of how Dad worked so hard to make our lives so miserable. Even when he refused to pay all he was supposed to pay for school, you worked extra just to make sure none of us missed out. I think the best thing you did was what you did not do. You never spoke bad about Dad. You never told me he had other "new" kids to support; he did.
>
> With all my love, I thank you for not raising us in a home where the other parent was the bad one, like with my friends who went through divorces. Dad is and has been a jerk, I know it, not because of you, but because he chose to be. I do love you both (you would probably still slap my behind if I said I didn't love Dad), but I love, respect and admire you more than anybody on the face of the earth.
>
> Love,
>
> John

Barbara beamed at me. And we both knew it had been worth it.

Robert A. Concolino

Our Christmas Boy

As an only child, Christmas was a quiet affair when I was growing up. I vowed that some day I'd marry and have six children, and at Christmas my house would vibrate with energy and love.

I found the man who shared my dream, but we had not reckoned on the possibility of infertility. Undaunted, we applied for adoption and, within a year, he arrived.

We called him our Christmas Boy because he came to us during that season of joy, when he was just six days old. Then nature surprised us again. In rapid succession, we added two biological children to the family—not as many as we had hoped for, but compared with my quiet childhood, three made an entirely satisfactory crowd.

As our Christmas Boy grew, he made it clear that only he had the expertise to select and decorate the Christmas tree each year. He rushed the season, starting his gift list before we'd even finished the Thanksgiving turkey. He pressed us into singing carols, our frog-like voices contrasting with his musical gift of perfect pitch. Each holiday he stirred us up, leading us through a round of merry chaos.

Our friends were right about adopted children not

being the same. Through his own unique heredity, our Christmas Boy brought color into our lives with his irrepressible good cheer, his bossy wit. He made us look and behave better than we were.

Then, on his twenty-sixth Christmas, he left us as unexpectedly as he had come. He was killed in a car accident on an icy Denver street, on his way home to his young wife and infant daughter. But first he had stopped by the family home to decorate our tree, a ritual he had never abandoned.

Grief-stricken, his father and I sold our home, where memories clung to every room. We moved to California, leaving behind our friends and church.

In the seventeen years that followed his death, his widow remarried; his daughter graduated from high school. His father and I grew old enough to retire, and in December 1986, we decided to return to Denver.

We slid into the city on the tail of a blizzard, through streets ablaze with lights. Looking away from the glow, I fixed my gaze on the distant Rockies, where our adopted son had loved to go in search of the perfect tree. Now in the foothills there was his grave—a grave I could not bear to visit.

We settled into a small, boxy house, so different from the family home where we had orchestrated our lives. It was quiet, like the house of my childhood. Our other son had married and begun his own Christmas traditions in another state. Our daughter, an artist, seemed fulfilled by her career.

While I stood staring toward the snowcapped mountains one day, I heard a car pull up, then the impatient peal of the doorbell. There stood our granddaughter, and in her gray-green eyes and impudent grin, I saw the reflection of our Christmas Boy.

Behind her, lugging a large pine tree, came her mother,

stepfather and ten-year-old half-brother. They swept past us in a flurry of laughter; they uncorked wine and toasted our homecoming. They decorated the tree and piled gaily wrapped packages under the boughs.

"You'll recognize the ornaments," said my former daughter-in-law. "They were his. I saved them for you."

When I murmured, in remembered pain, that we hadn't had a tree for seventeen years, our cheeky granddaughter said, "Then it's time to shape up."

They left in a whirl, shoving one another out the door, but not before asking us to join them the next morning for church and for dinner at their home.

"Oh," I began, "we just can't."

"You sure as heck can," ordered our granddaughter, as bossy as her father had been. "I'm singing the solo, and I want to see you there."

We had long ago given up the poignant Christmas services, but now, under pressure, we sat rigid in the front pew, fighting back tears.

Then it was solo time. Our granddaughter's magnificent soprano voice soared, dear and true, in perfect pitch. She sang "O Holy Night," which brought back bittersweet memories. In a rare emotional response, the congregation applauded in delight. How her father would have relished that moment.

We had been alerted that there would be a "whole mess of people" for dinner—but thirty-five! Assorted relatives filled every corner of the house; small children, noisy and exuberant, seemed to bounce off the walls. I could not sort out who belonged to whom, but it didn't matter. They all belonged to one another. They took us in, enfolded us in joyous camaraderie. We sang carols in loud, off-key voices, saved only by that amazing soprano.

Sometime after dinner, before the winter sunset, it occurred to me that a true family is not always one's own flesh and blood. It is a climate of the heart. Had it not been for our adopted son, we would not now be surrounded by caring strangers who would help us hear the music again.

Later, our granddaughter asked us to come along with her. "I'll drive," she said. "There's a place I like to go." She jumped behind the wheel of the car and, with the confidence of a newly licensed driver, zoomed off toward the foothills.

Alongside the headstone rested a small, heart-shaped rock, slightly cracked, painted by our artist daughter. On its weathered surface she had written, "To my brother, with love." Across the crest of the grave lay a holly-bright Christmas wreath. Our number-two son, we learned, sent one every year.

As we stood by the headstone in the chilly but somehow comforting silence, we were not prepared for our unpredictable granddaughter's next move. Once more that day her voice, so like her father's, lifted in song, and the mountainside echoed the chorus of "Joy to the World," on and on into infinity.

When the last pure note had faded, I felt, for the first time since our son's death, a sense of peace, of the positive continuity of life, of renewed faith and hope. The real meaning of Christmas had been restored to us. Hallelujah!

Shirley Barksdale

Judy's Birthday

It was a high counsel that I once heard given to a young person, "Always do what you are afraid to do."

Ralph Waldo Emerson

I'm not sure exactly how or when Judy and I met. All I do know is that when she entered my life, a ray of sunshine broke through the clouds. At a time when my world was shrinking, Judy saw the opposite possibilities and gave me the spark I needed to create a new life . . . a life after multiple sclerosis.

In 1979, I was diagnosed with primary progressive MS. It wasn't long until I began retreating from all but essential family activities. My energy level was poor. Getting dressed required a two-hour nap. When I could no longer stand up on my own or move myself from place to place, I was devastated. The things I could do for myself were dwindling. My world shrank smaller and smaller by the day. By 1984, I was using a scooter full time because I had no use of my legs or dominant right hand and arm.

But all these changes in my life didn't scare Judy off, as

it did some of my friends. She didn't care that I couldn't baby-sit her kids or take my turn driving carpool. She just cared about me and what I was going through.

One of the many things Judy did for me was to encourage me to write. Before raising her own children, she was an English teacher. After reading a couple of things I wrote, Judy saw something that I didn't see: that I could write. She mentored me and cajoled me through years of self-doubt. Her gentle prodding was always sensitive and understanding. She could see the toll MS was taking on my life. But she didn't give up on me. So many times she'd help lift me up when I was down. She gave me hope that there was still something important I could do.

It was not surprising that Judy had a wonderful circle of friends, and those friends also accepted me. When Judy was about to turn forty-five years old, her friends wanted to celebrate in a special way. They wanted to drive from our hometown of Madison, Wisconsin, to Milwaukee for lunch and meet two other friends who had recently moved to Milwaukee. The girls wanted me to join them.

My initial response was to say I couldn't go. Milwaukee was an hour and a half from Madison, and I could never be gone from home that long without using the rest room. No one besides my husband, David, had ever helped me in the rest room before. And who would lift me in and out of the passenger seat of our full-size, wheelchair-accessible van, and help me into my scooter? Only David had ever done that. What if the restaurant everyone wanted to go to wasn't accessible? And most important, would I be able to handle a whole day of activity without my daily nap?

I'm usually a positive, upbeat person, but this time, I was afraid the adventure would be too much for me. Then Judy called. Her lilting Oklahoma twang always made me smile. She said it wouldn't be a party without me. They had selected a restaurant that was wheelchair accessible, and it had an accessible rest room. The girls had talked and would do anything necessary to help me, including helping me in the rest room. Wouldn't I please reconsider and come along?

For days, I vacillated between going and not going. Then, one by one, the girls called to talk to me about the birthday adventure. The more we talked, the more I began to believe that maybe I could do this. We had shared so much, the girls and I—births, deaths, marital problems, the challenges of raising children, and aging parents. For years, we had been each other's "family away from home." These women knew my limits and what they were offering. Why couldn't I accept it? Was my pride getting in the way?

For years I had been giving up pieces of my life. And once I gave something up, like working, driving, dressing myself, standing, it was gone forever. It never came back. Was this a chance to put something I had lost back in my life?

I think what tipped the balance was my love and respect for my friend Judy. This was something I could do for her. With everyone's help and encouragement, I was willing to take the risk and join in the celebration.

To prepare, I rested for days prior to the party. When the day arrived, Dave lifted me into the van passenger seat while the girls watched. Then he put the 110-pound Amigo scooter in the back storage area. We talked about how to get me out of the van in Milwaukee and then how to get me back in again for the ride home. Two or three of the women would help me with each of the transfers. Nobody was fazed. Their attitude was, "Tell us what we have to do, and we'll do it." We discussed how they would help me in the rest room. Two other women would help with that task. I was glad that everyone was sharing in helping me. I didn't ever want to be a burden to any one person.

With instructions given, my husband gave me a good-luck kiss, and we were off.

The trip to Milwaukee and the party were a huge success! We laughed, joked, reminisced and made new memories. I returned home tired but exhilarated. I'd had a wonderful time and that night cried tears of happiness because I had done something I *never thought* I'd be able to do. Giving myself permission to accept the help I needed was the single most important thing I could have done for myself.

It may have been Judy's birthday, but I was the one who received the greatest gift.

Shelley Peterman Schwarz

The Special Olympics

A couple of years ago, when I was going to college, I volunteered to be a finish-line "hugger" at the Kentucky Special Olympics held in Richmond. Because I was studying to become a special-education teacher, I was very interested in the games and the people and wanted to be more involved.

The day of the event dawned dreary, wet and gray. I arrived early and watched as the participants arrived with their families, friends and school groups. Even though it started to rain and a cold wind blew, I didn't hear a single person complain. In fact, most of the participants were so excited that they didn't seem to notice the weather at all.

When the sky cleared up a bit, the first games began. My job was to stand at the end of a lane on the track and hug the person in that lane when he or she crossed the finish line. It seemed to me that many of the participants completed their races just so they could get that "finish" hug. As the arms of the hugger closed around them, their faces lit up with pure joy, whether they came in first or dead last.

While we huggers stood around, waiting for one race to

end and the next to begin, we talked. I was told that most of the participants had been training for the races all year. I was impressed. A dedicated athlete, I had been captain of my high school soccer team for two years, but even *I* hadn't trained year-round.

I also noticed that, unlike many athletes today, the Special Olympic participants weren't there just to win. They didn't play dirty or talk negatively about the people they were racing against. In fact, they hugged and wished each other luck before they started, and hugged again when it was over, whether they had won or not. I even saw one boy offer his gold medal to the man next to him. The boy explained that even people who come in last place are winners, and after all, the man had worked just as hard as he had.

What I remember most vividly from that day was the long-distance race. It was a long race by any standards: twelve laps around the track. There were only four participants, three boys and one girl. They were only a couple of laps into the race when the rain started up again. Standing in the rain, I began to feel miserable. My feet hurt. I was soaking wet. I was hungry. I was cold when the rain and wind came and hot when the sun came out. I thought irritably: *This race is lasting entirely too long.* Even though the three boys were nearly finished, the girl was at least four laps behind. I wondered why she kept going when there was obviously no way she could win.

Finally, the three boys finished and the girl was running alone. The boys didn't go up for their award right away, but waited by the track, cheering the girl on each time she went by. *She is so far behind,* I thought. *Why doesn't she just quit?*

She was the runner in my lane, and each time she ran by me, I almost wished that she would just stop for her hug. She was wet and in pain and obviously exhausted.

As she completed each lap, her face was a little redder and she was holding her side just a little bit more. But she didn't quit.

By the time she finished the race, she was barely running. The audience went wild when she crossed the line. She fell into my arms and started crying. I thought to myself that she was crying because she was so wet and cold, or she hurt so badly, or she was embarrassed for taking so long. Then I heard her mumbling something into my shoulder. She pulled away, folded her hands and began to pray. "Thank you, dear God, for giving me the strength to finish the race today. Thank you for letting the boys win. Thank you for all of these nice people." She hugged me again and then made her way to the awards table.

I stood motionless, astonished and awed. I couldn't believe what I just heard. Tears coursed down my face as I watched her joyfully accept her award for fourth place.

At that moment, I understood why these Olympics were "special."

Denaé Adams

The Classified Ad

I noticed the woman by my desk immediately when I entered the newsroom. She wasn't sitting in my side chair, waiting; she was pacing back and forth, playing with her hands. When the secretary told me she wanted my help to write a classified ad, I was doubly intrigued. Our paper is small, but I'm a features writer; I don't usually sell ad space. And people who place ads to sell things like houses, cars or pianos usually do it over the phone. But as I was about to find out, people who place ads to sell themselves do it in person.

The ad that the woman wanted to place was to adopt a baby. It was very important to her that the wording be just right, so she had asked to speak to a writer. Of course, I'd seen ads in the big newspapers like the one she wanted to place, but our newspaper had not, as far as I knew, ever run one. Still, there are standard grab lines for these ads. I suggested several to her: *Wanted, Baby to Love; Please Give Us Hope;* or *Dear Birth Mother, Let Us Help You.* The ad would contain information about her and her husband—that they were stable, could afford to raise a child, and that they had a lot of love to give. We included a toll-free number that a birth mother could use at any hour of the day or night to contact the couple. What I tried to keep out of the copy was the desperation I could hear in this woman's voice.

I spent a lot of time with her. I could see how difficult this was for her. She looked to be about my age—in her early forties—and she kept twisting her wedding band nervously. When her eyes rested for a moment on the photo on my desk of my four daughters, she said, "You are so fortunate."

"I know," I answered. And then, because I didn't know what else to say, I said, "Maybe you will be, too." But then something occurred to me: The major newspapers carried ads like these often and their circulations were hundreds of times what ours was. Why, I wondered, didn't this woman try those papers?

"I already have," she said. "In fact, we've advertised everywhere and tried every imaginable avenue. My husband and I have really decided to stop trying. But I work close to here, and I decided on my way in this morning that one more ad wouldn't hurt. And who knows?" She smiled weakly, handed me a check to run the ad for three weeks and left.

I felt so sad for this woman. The news stories were always filled with adoption heartaches: People would go to foreign countries in search of adoptable children, only to meet with bureaucratic red tape. They would incur huge expenses, only to be duped by unscrupulous lawyers or baby brokers. Even if an adoption went well, through proper channels, there were court cases where the adoptive parents had to give up the baby when a birth parent changed his or her mind.

Yes, I was lucky. I glanced at the photo of my kids and went back to work.

A week later, the woman called. "Please don't run the ad again," she said. Something in her tone of voice made me dare to ask if she had good news.

"Yes," she said. "We've connected with a birth mother. The baby is due in a month!"

"That's great news!" I said. "I hope it all goes well." Then, because I'm a features writer, I asked her if she would keep in touch if her adoption experience turned out to have a happy ending. She agreed.

A month later, the woman called to tell me that she and her husband had a son. All had gone smoothly, but the adoption would not be final for six months. At the end of that time, she would feel comfortable giving me the story.

I thought about that woman many times over the next six months, particularly when a news story came across my desk that had anything to do with a child. And there were plenty of stories during that time period: The world's first set of living septuplets was born in Iowa. A Wisconsin couple was indicted on child abuse charges; they had kept their seven-year-old daughter in an animal cage in a dark, cold basement. A newborn was kidnapped from the nursery of a county hospital but found unharmed and returned to his mother.

All of these stories evoked strong emotion in me. But I had a personal involvement in the drama of this woman's adoption experience. I think I identified with her in some way. I couldn't imagine what my life would be like if I had been childless. I didn't want to try.

One winter afternoon, as I was bundling up to leave for the day, my mind on carpools and dinner, my phone rang. I recognized her voice immediately.

"The adoption is final!" she said. "I knew he was ours from the moment he was put into my arms, but now it's all legal and finished! Would you like to come and meet him?"

I was so happy to hear good news. I made an appointment with her for the next day. I also told her that I would bring a photographer with me and the newspaper would love to give her a free portrait.

When we arrived at her home, the baby was sleeping. The woman ushered us in and offered us refreshments. Everything in the house was lovely. The smell of cinnamon added to the coffee and the atmosphere. The fire crackled in the fireplace.

"His name is Ben," she said, as I started to take notes. "He slept through the night right from the start. Now he's smiling and starting to turn over. Of course, I'm not rushing him. I waited so long for this baby. If he's a little slow, it's okay with me." She paused. "Oh, I should tell you— Ben has Down's syndrome."

I stopped writing. I wasn't sure how to react. But the new mother smiled. "Ben was meant for us, don't you see? I've got plenty of time to help him and he needs me even more than a normally developing child would."

At that moment, the baby monitor on the coffee table told us that Ben was up. His mother went to get him. I could hear her crooning softly to him as she picked him up and changed him. And I could hear his contented cooing in response.

She sat on the sofa, holding her son. Both of them smiled as the photographer took the picture. "You wanted a story with a happy ending," said my new friend. "You got it."

As I put on my coat, took a last look around that house and watched her kiss the top of her son's head softly, I knew, without a doubt, she was right.

Marsha Arons

The Mop Angel

When my two-year-old son, Larkin, climbed onto my lap saying, "Mommy, my tummy hurts," I thought it was a relapse of the flu. In a way, I was even glad he had a fever because it gave me something concrete to do: give him Tylenol, remove his clothes and let him soak in a lukewarm bath. That's one universal thing about mommies: We're best when we're in charge, able to help, able to make everything all right.

But on that Friday in May 1992, everything wasn't all right. Not only was my youngest sick, the television was depicting rioting and burning in Los Angeles—only blocks from where my mother lived. Despite repeated attempts to reach her, the phone lines remained jammed.

After his bath, Larkin crawled back into my lap, moaning and burning. As the afternoon wore on, his fever continued to rise. The nurse on the telephone agreed it was probably the flu, but I should bring him in just to be safe. I loaded the other kids—eleven-year-old Robin, six-year-old Summer, five-year-old Emerald and four-year-old Jesse—into the car, and off we went.

Our pediatrician lost his smile as he examined Larkin's

hot little body. His gentle fingers pressed the boy's abdomen and the anguished moans continued. After a few moments of unnerving concentration, the doctor sent us across the street to the hospital emergency room. "Larkin is too young to have problems with his appendix," he reassured us.

The surgeon at the hospital also muttered something about it being "highly unusual" for a two-year-old to have appendicitis. But he wanted another opinion.

At this point, the only help I could give was to appear calm for the other children. It got harder and harder as time passed—ten minutes, twenty minutes, half an hour. By the time the next doctor arrived, Larkin's moaning had ceased and the toddler lay quiet and still. Despite IV fluids being pumped into him, his temperature continued to soar.

The surgeon's verdict was swift: My son needed surgery, immediately.

Before I could push any questions through the lump in my throat, the doctor was gone. A team of nurses began to prep Larkin for surgery. I tried to fight the chill in my heart as I called my husband.

He arrived while Larkin was still waiting. A resolutely analytical man, he is quickly overwhelmed in any sort of emotional crisis. I was grateful that he took the other children home for supper, but it was clear he couldn't get out of that hospital fast enough. I knew he couldn't face coming back.

So Larkin and I waited. And waited. A nurse rushed through to say an auto accident had filled the operating rooms, but we'd be next. Another half hour went by.

Between victims, a masked surgeon ran in to check Larkin. Above his mask, his forehead creased more deeply. Then he was gone.

For two more hours, we waited. The antibiotics were

losing. Larkin grew hotter. He lay motionless, his fingers clinging to mine. Occasionally, he opened glazed eyes to make sure I was still there. Then he faded back out.

Every parent's nightmare folded in around me. My child was going to die, and there was nothing I could do.

If only there was something I could do, or at least someone to cling to, the way my sick baby clung to me! Instead, I sat alone, praying and holding Larkin's burning hand, feeling every tick of the clock.

Please, God. Please, somebody.

At 2 A.M. the curtain flew back. "Okay. We've got an operating room. Let's go!" The gurney sped down the hall, my hand and my son's still linked as I raced beside him.

At the door to the operating room, I pried Larkin's fingers from mine and he half woke, terrified and screaming, "Mommy, Mommy!"

The doors swung shut behind him. The sound quivered in the hallway air.

In the waiting area, the television was on, continuing riot coverage showing blood and flames, the city of Los Angeles lost in fear and hatred; a city that held my mother in its furious grasp.

It was too much. I sat down on the floor. Terrified and completely powerless, I leaned against the wall and sobbed.

Dimly, I was aware that the elevator doors across from me chimed open. A wiry little cleaning lady emerged, pushing a big fuzzy dust mop. I turned my head away to hide my tears. There was a moment of silence, neither of us moving or speaking.

Then she leaned her mop against the wall and slid down beside me.

"So, who you got in there?" she asked, nodding her head at the O.R.

"My son," I gulped. The torrent of the day's emotions swept through me, and I found myself pouring out everything. Through the jerky stream of words and sobs, she sat holding one of my hands in her own rough, worn ones, muttering and patting me gently.

At last I was empty, tired, and oddly enough, no longer scared. I looked down at her hands on mine, noting what a hard life was reflected in hers.

She began to speak of her own children, one dead, one far away, the youngest on drugs. She'd raised them alone, did the best she could. Now she was raising her grand-daughter, too. As she spoke of how smart and precious this little girl was, her face softened. Her voice was quiet when she talked of the girl's mother, lost to a crack habit, beyond even a mother's help.

"But . . . you've had so many sorrows! It doesn't seem fair! How do you possibly survive and go on?"

She laughed off my indignation. "You just gotta have faith. Nothing lasts forever; it all passes on. And when you can't hold on no more, you just let go and let the angels carry your troubles awhile." She patted me again. "It'll be all right."

She stayed with me, sitting in silence, until the O.R. doors opened.

Dr. Taylor emerged, weary and smiling. "We got it," he said cheerfully. "Gangrenous, but it didn't rupture. He'll be fine."

As I followed the gurney to the recovery room, the elevator doors chimed open. I turned in time to see them slide closed on a wiry woman with a day's work yet ahead.

Larkin slept peacefully as the dark hours gave way to the first light of a new day. On the television, the images of hate had given over to images of prayer and repair, people joining together to heal rather than hurt. I knew instinctively what I would find out later that morning: My mother was safe.

Touching the fragile fingers of my son, I recalled the cleaning woman's words. How sometimes knowing how to be in charge is as important as knowing how to let go. I also believed what else she said: that when we can't hold on any longer, the angels will carry our troubles awhile. I smiled at the knowledge that sometimes these angels are human—and sometimes, just sometimes, they carry mops.

Lizanne Southgate

Grandma Is on Her Feet Again

Don't just count your years, make your years count.

Ernest Meyers

By July of 1996, I was in a nursing home, and my litany of woes would depress anyone: I had no legs, no sight in one eye, and the doctor had just announced I had to learn to give myself insulin to control my diabetes. I was seventy-seven years old, and it was clear my "up years" were over.

"It's okay, Mom," my daughters said. "We'll bring you home and care for you. We'll arrange for a nurse."

Be a burden to my daughters? Have them carry me everywhere because I couldn't move on my own? I cried myself to sleep every night.

In the nursing home, I had plenty of time to pray and think. The doctors had said I'd never walk again. But then, if I'd listened to everything that I'd been told, I wouldn't have had any "up years" at all! I smiled, remembering when I was a fifteen-year-old girl in Ireland, ready to board the ship to sail to America.

"You're so lucky, Margaret!" my friends chorused. "In America, the streets are paved with gold!"

Well, I never found gold on the streets, only a few pennies. But the can-do spirit in America fed my own will to make something of myself.

My first job was working in a hospital as a nurse's aide. I loved it, even though it meant being on my feet all day. What the heck? I had two strong legs. In fact, I enjoyed it so much, I devoted my life to hospital work.

Between work and family, life had sure been good back then. When I retired, I looked forward to my "golden years." But my health began to deteriorate. It seemed I was always going to my podiatrist with ulcers on my toes. I had one toe amputated and another was treated for gangrene. After an infection, the surgeon had to amputate my left leg. I was devastated. After seven months in the hospital, I went to a nursing home for rehabilitation. I was only there for three weeks—till May 1996—when I developed a black spot on my large right toe. Back in the hospital, the surgeon told me my right leg would have to come off.

I was depressed and cried for a week. What would I do with no legs? I had already lost the sight of my left eye. I was seventy-seven years old. By the time I ended up back in the nursing home in July 1996, I was ready to give up. It seemed that all around me were folks who'd lived their lives and packed in their hopes. They'd accepted their down years—some seemed to be just waiting to die.

But in a very odd way, having the doctors tell me I would never walk again resonated with voices from my past. Had I ever taken the easy way before? What if I'd stayed safe with what I knew in Ireland? What if I'd come to the United States and waited to find all that gold on the streets?

As I prayed each day, the message came strongly: "God

helps those who help themselves. Had my earlier 'up years' just happened?" a voice asked me.

No. I had been willing to work hard, to fight to make them happen. I saw clearly that this was what I'd need to do again. It wasn't a matter of age but determination.

I started by washing and dressing myself. I would let no one help me. The staff tried to tell me I was being too independent, but I was determined. Next, I taught myself to get in and out of bed.

My biggest battle came in insisting that the doctors give me permanent prosthetics. They said I was being foolish. I said, "Which way's the gym?"

My first day in the gym, I was so determined to walk that I took two steps, which amazed everyone. From that day on, I worked so hard that the other residents started telling me I was an inspiration to them.

In time, the staff was asking me to help others see what they could do, and I even gave lessons on how to get in and out of bed. In the hospital, I'd already learned how to drive my own wheelchair. Now I learned to walk with a walker. I asked my therapist to teach me to climb stairs and I practiced three times a day. My next challenge was learning to use the toilet without assistance. This was a major accomplishment, and I did it!

I went into the nursing home in July 1996 with no legs and no hope, and on February 23, 1997, I walked out! Not only that, but I was taken to my own home, where I could live independently. Along the way, I'd learned to ask for, and gratefully accept, the help and support of my doctors, therapists, nurses, aides and family.

I found it unexpectedly hard to leave all the friends I'd made in the nursing home. My family surprised me with business cards that read "Role Model Extraordinaire" to leave behind with the patients and staff, so they knew where to call me for a pep talk.

Not that I was at home much! Shortly after my release, I traveled to Virginia with my daughter and son-in-law for my granddaughter's wedding. On the way there, we made several stops to go sightseeing. I can't describe the thrill of simply being able to get in and out of the Jeep, being a whole person. Being part of the human race again!

That was a wonderful time, being together with my whole family, including six grandchildren and three greats! But almost as exciting is waking up every day, knowing I can get in and out of the shower by myself, cook and go out on my Rascal scooter.

Hallelujah! The "up years" are back.

Margaret McSherry

8

SPECIAL MOMENTS

When your life is filled with the desire to see the holiness in everyday life, something magical happens: Ordinary life becomes extraordinary, and the very process of life begins to nourish your soul!

Rabbi Harold Kushner

The Department Store Santa

"Why are there so many different Santas?" I asked my mother, tightly clutching her hand as we walked along the icy downtown sidewalk. I was five years old.

"They're all Santa's helpers," my mother answered. "The *real* Santa is the one at Leavitt's department store. You met him last year, remember?"

I nodded, not doubting for a moment that he was genuine. The Santas everywhere else, with their scraggly cotton beards, heavily rouged cheeks and drooping, padded bellies bore little resemblance to the Santa in my favorite picture book, *The Night Before Christmas.* But the Santa at Leavitt's department store—well, he looked as if he had just stepped right off one of the pages.

"Can we go see Santa today?" I asked. "Please?"

"Next week," my mother answered, glancing at her watch. "I promise."

But five days later, instead of visiting Santa, I found myself on a cold table in a doctor's examining room.

Wide-eyed, I stared at the doctor as he spouted a lot of medical terms I didn't understand . . . until he said, "She'll probably lose all of her hair."

"You're mistaken," my mother responded, shaking her head. "I don't want to offend you, but I'm going to take her to a specialist for a second opinion."

And she did. Unfortunately, the diagnosis was the same. I had a form of juvenile alopecia, a disease that would make my hair fall out.

I can remember watching my mother choking back tears every time she found a clump of my blonde curls lying on the floor or scattered across my pillowcase. I also remember angrily refusing to believe her when she assured me that my hair would grow back.

Understandably, I didn't have much Christmas spirit that year. Although I felt fine physically, the sight of myself pale and bald made me want to lock myself in my room and hide under my bed. When my father enthusiastically invited me on our annual father-daughter shopping spree to buy Christmas gifts for my mother—an event I'd always looked forward to—I told him I didn't want to go.

But Dad could be persuasive when he wanted to be. He convinced me that without my help and suggestions, he probably would end up buying my mother the most hideous Christmas gifts in the history of the world.

Solely for the sake of salvaging my mother's Christmas, I agreed to go shopping with him.

Downtown, the throngs of shoppers, cheerful Christmas music and thousands of twinkling lights made me temporarily forget my problems. I actually began to have a good time . . . until Dad and I decided to stop for a cup of hot cocoa.

"Hi, Lou!" one of the customers greeted my father when we walked into the coffee shop. "Say, I didn't know you had a little boy! I thought you only had a daughter."

I burst into tears.

My father quickly ushered me out of the coffee shop and led me toward Leavitt's department store. "I have just the thing to cheer you up," he said, forcing a smile. "A visit with Santa! You'd like that, wouldn't you?"

Sniffling, I nodded.

But even as I stood in line in Leavitt's toy department, where Santa sat on a regal, red velvet throne trimmed in gold, my tears wouldn't stop. When my turn finally came, I shyly lowered my head and climbed onto Santa's lap.

"And what's your name?" Santa asked kindly.

Still not looking up, I carefully pronounced my full name—first, middle and last—just to make certain he would be able to find my house on Christmas Eve.

"And what would you like Santa to bring you for Christmas?" he asked.

My tear-filled eyes met his. Slowly I removed my brown stocking cap and revealed my naked scalp. "I want my hair back," I told him. "I want it to be long and beautiful, all the way down to the floor, just like Rapunzel's."

Santa cast a questioning look at my father and waited for his nod before he answered. "It takes a long time for your hair to grow, sweetheart," Santa said. "And I'm very, very sorry, but even Santa can't speed things up. You'll have to be patient and never lose faith. Your hair will grow back in time; I promise you it will."

With all my heart, I believed his promise. And ten months later, when my hair did grow back, I was convinced it was due solely to Santa's magic.

The years passed, and when I graduated from high school, I went to work full time as a switchboard operator at Leavitt's department store. All my coworkers were friendly, but one employee in particular went out of his way to make me feel welcome. He was a retired professional boxer named "Pal" Reed, the store's handyman and jack-of-all-trades.

Pal had a knack for sensing when an employee was depressed, and he did everything he could to help. When

I was learning how to work the switchboard and became so frustrated over my mistakes that I was ready to quit, Pal bought me a box of chocolates to lift my spirits. He was so easy to talk to, I felt as if I had known him for years.

During my first Christmas season at Leavitt's, I went down to the stockroom one afternoon to get some gift boxes. There, standing in a corner with his back toward me, was the store's Santa, getting ready for his annual arrival in the store's toy department.

"I'm sorry," I said, embarrassed that I had interrupted him while he was dressing. "I didn't mean to barge in on you."

Santa quickly put on his beard before he turned to face me, but no beard or long white wig could conceal his identity. He was the same Santa I had told my Christmas wish to fourteen years before.

He was Pal Reed.

He smiled knowingly at me, then softly said, "I remembered you the minute I heard your name—and I've never been more thrilled to see such a beautiful head of hair."

Sally A. Breslin

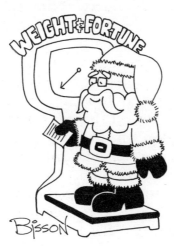

"You are fat, jolly and love children."

Reprinted by permission of Randy Bisson.

Halloween Angels

On Halloween, I brought my wife home from the hospital to live out her remaining days. Remembering that the children would come for trick-or-treat, and realizing I was not prepared with any candy, I quickly gathered whatever I could find in the house.

The first arrivals were three girls about fifteen years old. I apologized for my poor treats and told them I was not able to get any because of my wife's illness. They thanked me and went off. About a minute later they returned, and each one gave me a handful of candy from their bags. Through my tears, I tried to return it, but these wonderful young ladies rushed off, leaving me with: "We hope she gets well."

I do not know these beautiful young women, but I'd like them to know that their simple act of kindness brought joy and hope to me when there was none.

Even though my wife has since passed on, the memories of a sad time will be brightened by the thought of the kindness of these three angels. May God bless them.

Steven J. Lesko Jr.
Submitted by Laurie S. Brooks

Lucky Pennies

The cream of enjoyment in this life is always impromptu. The chance walk; the unexpected visit; the unpremeditated journey; the unsought conversation or acquaintance.

Fanny Fern

I grew up across the street from Mr. Kirby. He was a tall, thin, seventy-ish man who lived alone and apparently had no family and no visitors, except for the Meals-on-Wheels guy twice a week. During the summers, I would see Mr. Kirby taking his morning walk around the neighborhood. I would run to catch up with him so we could talk. He was the only adult I knew who talked to me as if I was a person, and not just some silly eight- or nine-year-old girl. Once, he told me he didn't have any grandchildren, and asked me if I'd like to be his surrogate granddaughter. After I received a complete definition of the word "surrogate," I gladly accepted.

We would walk and talk for what seemed hours, almost every day. He told me about his wife (his high school sweetheart) who had died several years before. He told me stories about the war, though I was never sure which one. He did magic tricks like pulling a quarter out of my ear. I used to check my ears for more change when I got home. On Saturday afternoons, Mr. Kirby would walk with me to the convenience store around the corner and let me pick out a dollar's worth of candy or gum or ice cream or whatever I wanted. I always tried to get it as close as I could to a dollar without going over. One day, I managed to gather up ninety-seven cents worth of bubble gum. As we walked away from the store, Mr. Kirby tossed the three pennies in change over his shoulder. I heard them clink on the hot asphalt parking lot.

"Mr. Kirby, why did you throw those pennies away?" I asked.

"To give someone a lucky day," he said.

"Oh, I know: 'See a penny, pick it up, and all the day you'll have good luck'—right?"

"You know," he said, "those who find lucky pennies need them the most because they are always looking down. Sometimes I'll take the shiniest penny I can find and drop it on the road in front of my house, just so I can watch it bring luck to someone's day."

"My mom says it's bad luck to be superstitious, Mr. Kirby." I admonished him with a serious tone and pretended to know what I was saying. He let out a roar of laughter and even slapped his knee. We had to stop walking for a moment so he could catch his breath. I stood there, holding my bag of gum, staring at him and trying to figure out what was so darn funny. I don't think he ever explained it.

As we began to walk again, he said, "You see, if you spend more time looking up and straight ahead, you don't need luck because you have confidence; you have optimism." He defined confidence and optimism and told me that I had both, and warned me never to lose them. I was too young then to know how hard it would be to hold onto those things; I was too young then to take much to heart. All I knew was that I had confidence, optimism, a brand-new bag full of bubble gum and a neighbor who regularly tossed pennies.

As the years went by, my life became busy, and I only had time to wave at Mr. Kirby as he sat on his front-porch swing. Sometimes I felt a twinge of what I identified later as guilt that I was running off here and there, while my surrogate grandfather, my former walking and talking partner, could only sit and wave good-bye. Usually, though, I didn't give much thought to Mr. Kirby or our friendship. I was preoccupied with school activities, friends, football games and football players. I know now that I did feel a sense of comfort in the very back of my mind knowing he was still there, always there, across the street, anytime I needed him.

After I went off to college, my friendship with Mr. Kirby became a vague memory. I was a defiant, independent young woman. I needed no one. I was cool. I feigned an air of confidence. I eschewed optimism. Optimism was for the cheerleaders and the Prozac crowd. My attitude attracted similar negative-minded people. We were wild and free. College classes were mere annoyances to endure between parties. I found several lucky pennies over those years. But no luck ever seemed to come my way.

Every year when I'd go home for Christmas, my mother would beg me to go visit Mr. Kirby. "He still talks about you and asks how you're doing. He would just love to see you," she'd say. I never made the time to cross the street. I think I was ashamed at whom I hadn't become, at what I wasn't. I never admitted that to myself then, but in my heart, I knew I was a better person than I had made myself out to be. Eventually, the superficial friendships faded. I never missed them.

After graduation, I went home for some job interviews. To my surprise, there was old Mr. Kirby sitting in his porch swing. He waved at me. "That you?" he yelled.

"Yes, Mr. Kirby, it's me," I responded, as I crossed the street and headed for his walkway.

"My, my, didn't you grow up to be a beautiful woman! And smart, too. I hear you just graduated from college! How 'bout we walk down to the corner store for a dollar's worth of candy?" He winked and slapped his knee. His false teeth sparkled the most genuine smile I'd seen in years. "Lordy, girl, you have the world at your doorstep. I always knew you'd be a success. Imagine that, a grand-daughter of mine so smart and successful!" He laughed the same hearty laugh of almost fifteen years before.

We sat in that swing and talked for hours. It was as if he hadn't aged at all. In fact, he seemed younger. And not nearly as tall. I had grown up in spite of myself. Just as I was feeling so grown up, I heard my mother calling me as she had when I was little. "Are you still over there? It's time for dinner." I gave Mr. Kirby a long hug and then held his hands tightly in mine. I didn't realize until that moment how important he was to whom I had become, and to whom I would be.

As I left the next morning for my first job interview, I'd like to say I found a shiny lucky penny, but I missed it. I was looking up.

Jill Williford Mitchell

Let Our Requests Be Known

Service had started, and the minister began his sermon in our small country church in southeastern North Carolina. Everyone's attention was on the intense words being delivered to us that would feed us for the week and enlighten us on God's word.

Because our church was so small, there was no nursery. This gave me the privilege of having my active three-year-old daughter sit with her father and me. Along with being active, Tammie had a gift for words—that is, speaking them—and had not yet mastered the art of understanding that quietness was of the utmost importance in church, especially when the Sunday morning sermon was being delivered!

After many admonishments to be quiet, Tammie's father picked her up to take her outside for a little conference.

This was not the first time such an event had taken place, and she understood its significance. She also obviously understood the significance of prayer!

For as her father picked her up and was walking down the aisle to carry her outside, Tammie reached over his shoulders with her arms outstretched to the congregation and the minister. She then proceeded to call out to all who would listen, "Ya'll pray for me!"

Needless to say, it was a few minutes later before we could get back on track with the sermon.

Guess it proves we are never too young to "let our requests be known"!

Donna Kay Heath

Christmas in the Silver Egg

The spur of delight comes in small ways.

Robert L. Stevenson

My husband Dave and I have always believed you're never really poor as long as you have hope. And hope was about the only thing we had in the winter of 1948, when we packed up our little boys and left our family and friends in Oklahoma for the "boom town" of Houston, Texas, where we'd been told the streets were paved with jobs.

Knowing that better days were on the way, we cheerfully moved into a trailer court because it was the cheapest place we could find, and we rented the cheapest trailer in the court. It cost thirty dollars a month—inexpensive even by the standards of the times—and we christened it "the Egg" because it was shaped like a silver egg. At times, it didn't seem much bigger than an egg, either, especially with two active toddlers—Mike, age two, and Tony, three and a half. That made four of us trying to live in a teensy trailer not big enough to swing a cat in.

There was only one room in the Egg, and that room

served as dining room, kitchen and bedroom; the bathroom was as large as a broom closet. The bed was the size of a train bunk . . . maybe. David and I had to sleep in each other's arms every night, even if we were mad. But we didn't get mad too often—you can't cuddle up to someone like that without feeling loving, so I figured it was good for our marriage.

Because the boys were so little, we could all four squeeze into the breakfast nook—two seats facing each other, with a table between—if we really scrunched together. At night, that little table collapsed, and the boys slept on top of it.

A full-sized adult could touch from wall to wall if he stood with his arms outstretched. No one did, though, because the Egg wasn't grounded very well, and any time you touched a wall you were in for a shock. Literally. We all learned to walk around leaning inward.

Still, we managed to have a pretty good time. The trailer court was full of nice people and some of them were eccentric enough to delight me. One woman, who became one of my best friends, worked as a hula dancer in a carnival. She tacked her old grass skirts up at her window, parted them in the middle, tied them back, and presto—curtains!

"Isn't that a cute idea?" she asked proudly. I nodded, not daring to trust my voice because I was so full of the giggles.

So it was sort of fun, usually. Then Christmas drew near.

Houston Decembers aren't your snowy, Christmas-card kind of Decembers, but they can be very nice—delightfully warm with brilliant sunshine and even flowers and green grass. Or they can be miserable—chilly rain, gray skies and gloom. That's the kind of Christmas we had that year.

My background is Cherokee, and never before had I so missed my loving, extended family. Our Christmases in

Oklahoma might not have been opulent, but they were rich in love, laughter, savory smells of cooking and the earthy aroma of pine filling the house.

The trailer court was a sea of mud that clung to our shoes and came off on the floor the minute we stepped inside. Everything was damp, moldy and cold. Christmas seemed a million years away, but it was only a few days away—and there wasn't any money.

Oh, there was a wee bit. David had a job in a car lot—not selling, just washing the cars and shifting them around the lot. We didn't miss any meals, though the menu was mostly macaroni and cheese. But when David and I sat down four days before Christmas, we found that, even though we'd saved like crazy, we had less than ten dollars to provide Christmas dinner and gifts for two little boys.

"I guess there isn't going to be any Christmas this year, hon," David said, and for once, his brown eyes weren't sparkling. "No toys for the kids or anything."

Or anything. No grandparents, aunts, uncles and cousins bustling around, laughing and telling tales. No turkey on the carving board or special desserts mounded on the table.

No Christmas tree. In a way, that was the hardest thing for me. The Christmas tree had always been for me the very symbol of Christmas, of love and prosperity. Of hope.

Not that a tree could fit in the Egg, anyhow.

I clung to David a second longer than usual when he started off to work. My smile was very stiff, for it was rigidly holding back a sob.

That afternoon, the misting rain let up for the first time in days, so I took the kids for a walk. It was rough keeping a couple of little widgets cooped up in something like the Egg.

The wind was raw. We slogged through the mud, frosty hands clasped in each other's. My heart felt as mired as my feet—but Tony and Mike were having a wonderful time. After being shut inside for a couple of days, the outdoors was newly wonderful—especially because Christmas decorations were up all over! The boys splashed through the puddles and laughed with glee as they pointed out wreaths, plastic Santas and Christmas trees in windows.

Suddenly, Tony pointed at the far end of the trailer court. "Look, Mommy, look! A million Christmas trees. Come on, Mommy!"

Mike caught the excitement, and he and Tony towed me along like a couple of tug boats towing a shabby scow.

There weren't a million trees. It was actually a modest little lot, but the trees had been stuck into the ground so they looked like a small forest. The kids and I walked between them. Fir and pine, smelling wet and cold and fresh-smelling like Christmas! The earthy aroma took me back to my childhood Christmases, and my own excitement started building.

Then Tony whispered urgently, "Buy one, Mommy. Buy one now!"

And reality crashed down. There would be no tree for us. It just wasn't fair! They weren't so terribly expensive, but even the cheapest was beyond me. And all around, people were happily picking out this one or that. They were even fussy because the trees weren't absolutely perfect, so they'd ask the lot owner to trim off branches to make them look more symmetrical. How spoiled they were to ask that precious branches be cut off and just thrown away, when I longed so much for just . . .

My mouth dropped open ". . . for just one big, beautiful branch," I whispered. Yes, a big branch with a lot of little limbs would look almost like a miniature Christmas tree. In fact, even the smallest tree would be too big for the Egg, but a branch would be just right! Surely I could afford a branch!

I went over and pulled on the owner's sleeve. "How much would a branch cost?" I asked, feeling shy but fierce.

The man, chilled and seeing his trees like a little forest of dollar signs—he probably didn't have much money himself—snarled at me. "Lady, I don't sell branches. You want a tree, buy one. I ain't gonna cut one up just so you can have a branch."

My feelings weren't even hurt. "No, no!" I cried. "I don't want you to cut a branch from a tree. I want one of those." I pointed to the sizable pile of trimmed-off branches.

"Oh, sure," he grunted. "Them. Help yourself."

"How much for a big one?"

"Lady, I told you, I don't sell branches. Take all you want free."

I could hardly believe it! Joy overtook us as the boys and I hunkered down, selecting a branch with all the care that others were taking to pick out a full tree. When we were certain we'd found the most beautiful branch of all, we proudly carried it home, Mike holding the top, Tony holding the bottom, and me supporting the middle.

While my friend with the hula skirt baby-sat, I ran five blocks to the five-and-ten-cent store. I hid my packages when I got home. Then I retrieved the kids, and we anchored the branch firmly in one corner of the trailer, where it fit exactly. In the Egg, it looked as big as a real Christmas tree.

When David got home, we all decorated it together with a big package of tinsel I'd found for ten cents and some little balls really meant to decorate packages that had cost another dime. When we were done, it was—well, beautiful, that's all. David made a star out of the tinfoil from a found cigarette pack, and we perched it right up at the top. There weren't any lights, but it gleamed and glistened all by itself.

On Christmas Eve, David came home with a fat boiling hen he'd managed to buy for a dollar. She was cheap because she was tough, but no matter. I would boil her and boil her until she became tender, and David would make German dumplings to drop in the rich broth, just like his mother had taught him. He was a wonderful cook.

As that old hen boiled merrily away on the hot plate and the kids were cuddled down asleep on their table-bed, we put toys under the branch—two cars, two trucks, a fire engine and a red and yellow train. All plastic, all less than a quarter, but they looked wonderful. The trailer looked wonderful.

I reached up and kissed David's cheek. Although he was so tall, it was easy to reach him, for of course in the Egg, he was a little bent over. "There once were four people who lived in an Egg," I said.

"Oh, hon, hon!" He put his arm around me and pulled me close. His eyes were twinkling again like dark brown stars, and we stood together in the shadow of our tree, which smelled of Christmas and of magic, of the memory of childhood and of the promise of the future. Of hope.

And we knew we were one of the richest families on earth.

Mechi Garza

A Coke and a Smile

That man is richest whose pleasures are cheapest.

Henry David Thoreau

I know now that the man who sat with me on the old wooden stairs that hot summer night over thirty-five years ago was not a tall man. But to a five-year-old, he was a giant. We sat side by side, watching the sun go down behind the old Texaco service station across the busy street. A street that I was never allowed to cross unless accompanied by an adult, or at the very least, an older sibling. An unlikely pair, we sat together, perched on the top step. His legs reached down two stairs; mine dangled, barely reaching the first. The night was muggy and the air thick. It was the summer of 1959.

Cherry-scented smoke from Grampy's pipe kept the hungry mosquitoes at bay while gray, wispy swirls danced around our heads. Now and again, he blew a smoke ring and laughed as I tried to target the hole with my finger. I, clad in a cool summer nightie, and Grampy, in his sleeveless T-shirt, sat watching the traffic, trying to catch the elusive breeze. We counted cars and tried to guess the color of the next one to turn the corner. I was luckier at this game than Grampy.

Once again, I was caught in the middle of circumstances. The fourth born of six children, it was not uncommon that I was either too young or too old for something. This night I was both. While my two baby brothers slept inside the house, my three older siblings played with friends around the corner, where I was not allowed to go. I stayed with Grampy, and that was okay with me. I was where I wanted to be. My grandfather was baby-sitting while my mother, father and grandmother went out.

"Thirsty?" Grampy asked, never removing the pipe from his mouth.

"Yes," was my reply.

"How would you like to run over to the gas station there and get yourself a bottle of Coke?"

I couldn't believe my ears. Had I heard right? Was he talking to me? On my family's modest income, Coke was not a part of our budget or diet. A few tantalizing sips was all I had ever had, and certainly never my own bottle.

"Okay," I replied shyly, already wondering how I would get across the street. Surely Grampy was going to come with me.

Grampy stretched his long leg out straight and reached his huge hand deep into the pocket. I could hear the familiar jangling of the loose change he always carried. Opening his fist, he exposed a mound of silver coins. There must have been a million dollars there. He instructed me to pick out a dime. I obeyed. After he deposited the rest of the change back into his pocket, he stood up.

"Okay," he said, helping me down the stairs and to the curb, "I'm going to stay here and keep an ear out for the babies. I'll tell you when it's safe to cross. You go over to the Coke machine, get your Coke and come back out. Wait for me to tell you when it's safe to cross back."

My heart pounded. I clutched my dime tightly in my sweaty palm. Excitement took my breath away.

Grampy held my hand tightly. Together we looked up the street and down, and back up again. He stepped off the curb and told me it was safe to cross. He let go of my hand and I ran. I ran faster than I had ever run before. The street seemed wide. I wondered if I would make it to the other side. Reaching the other side, I turned to find Grampy. There he was, standing exactly where I had left him, smiling proudly. I waved.

"Go on, hurry up," he yelled.

My heart pounded wildly as I walked inside the dark garage. I had been inside the garage before with my father. My surroundings were familiar. My eyes adjusted, and I heard the Coca-Cola machine motor humming even before I saw it. I walked directly to the big old red-and-white dispenser. I knew where to insert my dime. I had seen it done before and had fantasized about this moment many times. I checked over my shoulder. Grampy waved.

The big old monster greedily accepted my dime, and I heard the bottles shift. On tiptoes I reached up and opened the heavy door. There they were: one neat row of thick green bottles, necks staring directly at me, and ice-cold from the refrigeration. I held the door open with my shoulder and grabbed one. With a quick yank, I pulled it free from its bondage. Another one immediately took its place. The bottle was cold in my sweaty hands. I will never forget the feeling of the cool glass on my skin. With two hands, I positioned the bottleneck under the heavy brass opener that was bolted to the wall. The cap dropped into an old wooden box, and I reached in to retrieve it. It was cold and bent in the middle, but I knew I needed to have this souvenir. Coke in hand, I proudly marched back out into the early evening dusk. Grampy was waiting patiently. He smiled.

"Stop right there," he yelled. One or two cars sped by me, and once again, Grampy stepped off the curb.

"Come on, now," he said, "run." I did. Cool brown foam sprayed my hands.

"Don't ever do that alone," he warned firmly.

"Never," I assured him.

I held the Coke bottle tightly, fearful he would make me pour it into a cup, ruining this dream come true. He didn't. One long swallow of the cold beverage cooled my sweating body. I don't think I ever felt so proud.

There we sat, side by side, watching the sun go down behind the old Texaco service station across the busy street. A street I had been allowed to cross by myself. Grampy stretched his long legs down over two stairs. I dangled mine, a bit closer to the first step this time, I'm sure.

Jacqueline M. Hickey

Enduring Labor

The nurse approached him, smiling. "The labor is going great," she said. "Wouldn't you like to come in?"

"Oh, no." The man shook his head.

The nurse returned to the mother's side, and the labor progressed smoothly. As the birth neared, the nurse returned to the man, now pacing frantically in the hall. "She's doing so well," she assured him. "Wouldn't you like to at least come in and see her?"

The man seemed to hesitate slightly, then shook his head again. "No, no, I couldn't do that." He jingled car keys in his sweaty palm and resumed his pacing.

The nurse went back into the room and coached Mom's valiant efforts in pushing the baby into the world. As the baby's head began to exit the birth canal, the nurse raced to the hall, grabbed the man by his elbow and dragged him to the bedside, saying, "You have got to see this!"

At that very moment, the baby boy was born and placed on the tummy of his mother, whose radiant smile shone through her tears. The man began to cry openly. Turning to the nurse, he sobbed, "You were right! This is the greatest moment in my life!"

By now, the nurse, too, was tearful. She put her arm around him, and he rested his head on her shoulder. She soothed, "No one should miss the birth of their son."

"This isn't my son," the man blubbered. "This isn't even my wife. I've never seen her before in my life. I was just bringing the car keys to my buddy across the hall!"

LeAnn Thieman

The Smile Behind the Tear

The doctor's words echoed in my head: "There's no need to bring her back; the chemotherapy is no longer working. She has three months at the most." Tears burned my eyes. Three months . . . that would be Easter.

I helped Momma get settled on the plane and then fastened her seat belt. I dropped into my place by the window, adjusted my sun shades, and stared out into the blowing rain—typical Houston weather.

I glanced sideways at Momma. Her head rested against the seat. I studied her familiar features, so comforting, such a part of me. I couldn't imagine life without Momma. I squeezed my soggy tissue and stared at the dark sky.

A light rustling caused me to look up as a tall young man brought a small girl, about seven years old, on board and sat her across from us.

"Have your mother call me as soon as you get home. You can come back in July and spend the summer with us." Stroking her hair, he whispered, "I love you, honey, and will miss you." Abruptly, he stood and almost ran from the plane.

I peeked through half-opened eyes at the child. A cute

kid with long blonde hair pulled back in a braid, big blue eyes, a little pug nose and one tooth missing. *Well, I hope she doesn't bother Momma.*

I clenched my fists and tried to push back the heavy, trapped feeling. *Three months,* I thought, *three months,* as we began our upward climb through the dreary sky.

The small girl, Lisa—that's what her name tag read—sat still, her head tilted. A big tear rolled down her chubby cheek, and she silently tried to conceal it.

Momma leaned over with a tissue and caught the tear. "Now where's the smile?" she asked.

Taken by surprise, Lisa's blue eyes opened wide. Before she could speak, a smile covered her face.

"There, I knew it would come." Momma settled back in the seat, her eyes still on the child. "Did you know that, Lisa? There is always a smile behind a tear."

Lisa shook her head. "How did you know that?"

"Oh, I just learned it through the years."

Yes, she had learned it through the years. My mind went back to those times long ago, from the early days when I skinned my knees to the teenage years when a boy broke my heart. As Momma wiped my tears, she softly spoke, "Let me tell you something, Cozy. There's a smile behind all these tears. Look at that knee. It will heal, and I bet you slow down the next time you run through that loose gravel."

Tears for a first love go even deeper, or I thought so at the time. "It'll hurt for a while," she whispered, as I sobbed into the darkness. She held my hand. "Life goes on, Cozy, and so will you." She had been right; I survived.

Now I watched Momma's face glow as she talked to Lisa. All of her life, she had been surrounded by children. She always had a story, a game and something to eat.

I turned back to the window and watched the dark clouds roll by. Yes, Momma knew about tears. How many nights during the last three years had she shed those tears so she would have that smile during the day?

Once again, I heard Lisa's voice. "I wish my mother and daddy would live together again, but they won't. Daddy is married, and Mother has a boyfriend."

I felt Momma move and heard her voice. "Sometimes people can't get along together and decide it's best to part. You want them to be happy, don't you?"

"Yes," Lisa answered, her voice trembling.

"How old are you, Lisa?"

"Almost seven."

"Let me tell you something, Lisa." Momma's weak voice seemed stronger. "These next years will fly by. Before you know it, you'll be out of school, out of college, and then you'll be married and have kids of your own."

Startled, Lisa looked up. "You're right, Miss . . . "? Her blue eyes questioned Momma for a name.

"Just call me Bessie."

"Okay, Miss Bessie," Lisa answered.

Momma continued, "Being separated from your parents isn't fun, so make the best of the time you share with each one. When you are with your father, love him, help him and try to get to know his wife." Momma dug around in her purse. "My throat gets dry, and this peppermint candy always seems to help. Here, you want a piece?"

I heard the rattle of cellophane paper and the child giggle. Then Momma began, "Your mother can be your best friend. A mother is someone special; she loves you no matter what. Don't be afraid to tell her your problems." All was quiet except the clicking of the candy.

"When you're grown, you'll have the love of two of the most important people in your life. You'll always have the happy memories of the time you spent with them."

My throat ached as I swallowed the scalding tears. I would have memories, a lifetime of happy memories.

"You'll have problems and lots of tears," Momma continued. "They come in everyone's life, but just remember: that smile will always follow." She patted Lisa's tiny foot propped on her seat. "Sometimes it might take longer because the problem is tougher, but take my word: the smile will come."

I gazed out the window. Bright rays of sun filled the sky as I dropped my sun shades into my purse. Smiling, I turned to Momma and kissed her cheek. "This one took a little longer."

The plane landed, and Lisa rose to leave. She turned back, exposing a snaggle-tooth smile. "Thank you, Miss Bessie, for sharing your candy and talking to me."

A twinge of guilt tugged at my heart. How could I have thought that this small child would be a bother to Momma? On a trying flight for both, they shared tears, comforting words, candy and smiles.

I felt as if a weight had been lifted from my body. I whispered, "Thank you, Miss Bessie, for talking to Lisa, and thank you, Momma, for talking to me."

Helen Luecke

The Not-So-White Christmas Gift

Through the front window of the drugstore where we both worked as assistant managers, I could see Lamar eagerly awaiting my arrival, his breath condensing on the glass as he peered out at me. A deal we had struck back in November had him working Christmas Day and me New Year's.

The weather outside was typical of Memphis at this time of the year. Lamar and I always hoped for a white Christmas, but this one had rolled by just like the previous twenty—cold and foggy, with nary a snowflake in sight.

As I pushed into the warmth of the store, Lamar looked relieved.

"Rough day?" I inquired.

Gesturing to the front cash register, Lamar moaned, "We had lines fifteen-deep yesterday. I've never seen so many people trying to buy batteries and film. Oh well, I guess that's one of the joys of working Christmas day."

"What do you want me to do today?" I asked.

"It will probably slow down around six tonight. The night after Christmas is usually dead. Then you can straighten this disaster of a toy aisle." He stooped to pick up a stray stuffed animal, which he shoved into my belly.

"And do something with this animal."

That little plush dog had become our Christmas mascot. We seemed to be forever picking it up off the floor. Five, maybe ten, times a day. It hadn't been a pretty toy to begin with. Now its long shaggy fur had become matted and soiled, as gray as the day outside, grimed with dust from the floor and dirt from the hands of children who had held it while their mothers waited for prescriptions to be filled. The toy had been marked down many times, without any takers. In that bright shiny world of Smurfs and Barbie dolls and G.I. Joes, I guess a little dog with dirty white fur just wasn't the plaything of choice. Still, every kid in Memphis must have squeezed that puppy at least once that Christmas season.

The afternoon bustled by with refunds, exchanges and the sale of half-price Christmas decorations, but at six o'clock, just as Lamar had predicted, business came to a halt. Out of sheer boredom, I went to work on the toy aisle. The first toy I encountered, of course, was that fluffy dog with the droopy ears, staring up at me from the floor one more time. I started to throw it away and write it off the inventory, but, I changed my mind and stuck it back on the shelf. Sentimental, I guess.

"Excuse me." A voice interrupted my deliberations. "Are you the manager?" I turned and saw a slender young woman with a little boy of five standing quietly beside her.

"I'm the assistant manager," I said. "How may I help you?"

The lady looked down for a moment, then put her chin up and said with something like a rasp in her voice, "My son hasn't had any Christmas. I was hoping you might have something marked down now. Something I could afford?"

I had grown cynical at the occasional homeless person's plea for quarters, but in her voice, I heard a note of sincerity and a pride that made her ache at having to ask such a question.

I looked down at the little boy, standing there so self-controlled in the midst of all those toys.

"I'm just marking the toys down now. What is it you're looking for?"

The young woman brightened, as though she had finally encountered someone who would listen. "I don't have much money, but I'd like to buy my son something special."

The boy's face lit up at his mother's words. Speaking directly to him, I said, "You pick out the best toy you could want for Christmas, okay?"

He glanced at his mother, and when she nodded her assent, he grinned ear to ear. I waited, curious to see which of the season's most popular toys he would choose. Maybe a race car set, or a basketball.

Instead, he walked right to that gruff old dog and hugged it as tightly as ever I had seen a kid clutch a toy. I acted as if I were brushing the hair out of my eyes, while I surreptitiously wiped away a tear.

"How much is that dog?" his mother asked, unfastening the clasp on a small, black coin purse.

"It's no charge," I said. "You'd be doing me a favor by taking it away."

"No, I can't do that," she insisted. "I want to pay for my son's Christmas present."

From the intense look in her eyes, I knew that she wanted to give her child a gift as much as he wanted to receive one.

"It's a dollar," I said.

She pulled a crumpled bill from her purse and handed it to me. Then she turned to her son and said, "You can take the dog home with you now. It's yours."

Once again I fumbled with the hair around my eyes, as the little boy beamed ecstatically. His mother smiled, too, and silently mouthed "Thank you" as they left the store.

Through the window, I watched them make their way into the Memphis evening. There still wasn't a snowflake in sight, but as I turned back to the toy aisle, I found, smiling, that I had gotten that old white-Christmas feeling after all.

Harrison Kelly

9

MIRACLES

*There are only two ways to live your life.
One is as though nothing is a miracle.
The other is as though everything is a miracle.*

It Happened on the Brooklyn Subway

Where there is great love there are always miracles.

Willa Cather

Marcel Sternberger, a native of Hungary, was a man of nearly fifty, with bushy white hair and kind brown eyes. A methodical man, he always took the 9:09 train from his suburban home to Queens, New York, where he caught a subway into the city.

On the morning of January 10, 1948, Sternberger boarded the 9:09 as usual. En route, he suddenly decided to visit a Hungarian friend who lived in Brooklyn and was ill.

So Sternberger changed to the subway for Brooklyn, went to his friend's house, and stayed until mid-afternoon. He then boarded a Manhattan-bound subway for his Fifth Avenue office. Here is Marcel's incredible story.

The car was crowded, and there seemed to be no chance of a seat. But just as I entered, a man sitting by the door suddenly jumped up to leave, and I slipped into his empty place.

I'd been living in New York long enough not to start conversations with strangers. But being a photographer, I have always had the peculiar habit of analyzing people's faces, and I was struck by the features of the passenger on my left.

He was probably in his late thirties, and when he glanced up, his eyes seemed to have a hurt expression in them. He was reading a Hungarian-language newspaper, and something prompted me to say in Hungarian, "I hope you don't mind if I glance at your paper."

The man seemed surprised to be addressed in his native language. But he answered politely, "You may read it if you like. I'll have time later on."

Instead of reading, we began to talk. During the half-hour ride to town, I learned his name was Bela Paskin. A law student when World War II started, he had been put into a German labor battalion and sent to the Ukraine. Later he was captured by the Russians and put to work burying the German dead. After the war, he covered hundreds of miles on foot until he reached his home in Debrecen, a large city in eastern Hungary.

When he went to his former address, he found the apartment that had once been occupied by his father, mother, brothers and sisters, as well as the apartment he had shared with his wife, were both occupied by strangers. None of them had ever heard of his family.

Full of sadness, he turned to leave when a boy ran after him, calling, *"Paskin bacsi! Paskin bacsi!"* That means "Uncle Paskin." The child was the son of some of his old neighbors. He went to the boy's home and talked to his parents. "Your whole family is dead," they told him. "The Nazis took them to Auschwitz."

Auschwitz had been one of the worst Nazi concentration camps. Hearing this, Paskin gave up all hope. A few days later, too heartsick to remain any longer in Hungary, he set out again on foot, stealing across border after border until he reached Paris. He managed to immigrate to the United States in October 1947, just three months before I met him.

The entire time he had been talking, I kept thinking that somehow his story seemed familiar. A young woman whom I had met recently at the home of friends had also been from Debrecen; she had been at Auschwitz; from there she had been transferred to work in a German munitions factory. Her relatives had been killed in the gas chambers. Later, she was liberated by the Americans and was brought here in 1946, in the first boatload of displaced persons.

Her story had moved me so much that I had written down her address and phone number, intending to invite her to meet my family and thus help relieve a little of the terrible emptiness in her life.

It seemed impossible that there could be any connection between these two people, but as I neared my station, I fumbled anxiously in my address book. I asked in what I hoped was a casual voice, "Was your wife's name Marya?"

He turned pale. "Yes!" he answered. "How did you know?"

He looked as if he were about to faint.

I said, "Let's get off the train." I took him by the arm at the next station and led him to a phone booth. He stood there like a man in a trance while I dialed her phone number.

It seemed a long time before Marya Paskin answered. (Later I learned her room was near the telephone, but she was in the habit of never answering it because she had few friends and the calls were always for someone else. This time, however, there was no one else at home, and after letting it ring for a while, she responded.)

When I heard her voice at last, I told her who I was and asked her to describe her husband. She seemed surprised at the question, but gave me a description. Then I asked her where she had lived in Debrecen, and she told me the address.

Asking her to hold the line, I turned to Paskin and said, "Did you and your wife live on such-and-such a street?"

"Yes!" Bela exclaimed. He was white as a sheet and trembling.

"Try to be calm," I urged him. "Something miraculous is about to happen to you. Here, take this telephone and talk to your wife!"

He nodded his head in mute bewilderment, his eyes bright with tears. He took the receiver, listened a moment to his wife's voice, then suddenly cried, "This is Bela! This is Bela!" and he began to mumble hysterically. Seeing that the poor fellow was so excited he couldn't talk coherently, I took the receiver from his shaking hands.

"Stay where you are," I told Marya, who also sounded hysterical. "I am sending your husband to you. We will be there in a few minutes."

Bela was crying like a baby and saying over and over again, "It is my wife. I go to my wife!"

At first I thought I had better accompany Paskin, lest the man should faint from excitement, but I decided that this was a moment in which no stranger should intrude. Putting Paskin into a taxicab, I directed the driver to take him to Marya's address, paid the fare, and said good-bye.

Bela Paskin's reunion with his wife was a moment so poignant, so electric with suddenly released emotion, that afterward neither he nor Marya could recall much about it.

"I remember only that when I left the phone, I walked to the mirror like in a dream to see if maybe my hair had turned gray," she said later. "The next thing I know, a taxi stops in front of the house, and it is my husband who comes toward me. Details I cannot remember; only this I know: that I was happy for the first time in many years.

"Even now it is difficult to believe that it happened. We have both suffered so much; I have almost lost the capability to not be afraid. Each time my husband goes from the house, I say to myself, 'Will anything happen to take him from me again?'"

Her husband is confident that no horrible misfortune will ever again befall them. "Providence has brought us together," he says simply. "It was meant to be."

Paul Deutschman

Take My Hand

The car crept slowly up the dark mountain road as February winds dusted the slick pavement with new-fallen snow. From the front seat, my two college friends navigated the old car over the icy road. I sat behind them with a broken seat belt.

The back end of the car fishtailed. "No problem, Mary," Brad reassured me, gripping the steering wheel. "Sam's house is just over the next ridge. We'll make it there safely."

I heaved a sigh. "I'm glad Sam's having a party. It'll be so good to see everyone again after Christmas break." I hoped my cheerful friends could bring me up from one of the lowest points of my life. Even Christmas at home in Hawaii had been disappointing, leaving my heart empty and hollow. Nothing had been the same since Dad died two years ago.

Sensing my despair, Dad's sisters had taken me aside after Christmas dinner. "Pray to the heavens, honey," they coaxed. "Your daddy is there. He can hear you and help you."

Pray? Bah, humbug, I thought, as I left the family gathering. *I've given up on God.*

Moonlight glistened off the icy pavement. Our car approached the bridge traversing the canal waters feeding the nearby lake. As we crossed the bridge, the car began swerving out of control. "Hang on!" Brad screamed. We spun 360 degrees before careening off the road. The car rolled over, slammed onto its top, and my body crashed through the rear window and onto the frozen earth. As I groaned, only half-conscious, I noticed no sounds from the front seat. I started crawling, hoping to find the road, and help. Digging my elbows into the ground, I dragged my battered body across the rough terrain. With the next pull, I slid over a knoll and somersaulted down the other side and into the freezing canal water.

The pain and cold left me limp. Then I heard a voice scream, "Swim!"

I began to stroke with my arms.

"Swim!" the voice called. It sounded like Dad. "Swim harder, Mary Ann!"

He was the only one who called me Mary Ann. "Daddy!" I cried, as the current pulled me under. I thrust myself through the surface of the water when I heard him scream again, "Swim harder!"

"Daddy, where are you? I can't see you!" I yelled, as the frigid waters pulled me under again.

Too frozen and weak to fight, I felt myself sinking deeper into the darkness. My head swayed back, and I gazed up through the surface of the water where a bright golden light glowed. Then I heard Daddy holler again, "Swim, Mary Ann! Take my hand!"

With all my might, I hurled my body upward, through the water and into the light. There, my daddy's hand extended. I recognized his touch, his grip as he pulled me up.

Then the light, the hand—the moment—vanished. I was clutching a chain extended across the canal.

"Daddy!" I cried. "Come back! Help me. Help me, Daddy!"

"Over here!" another voice yelled. "She's over here!" A stranger leaned toward the water's edge. "Hold on to the chain and pull yourself to shore!"

Hand over hand, I yanked my frozen torso within the stranger's reach, and he lifted me to the bank. My body and my mind were numb.

"Let's get you to the hospital," the man said, wrapping me in a blanket. He sniffed near my face. "Have you been drinking?"

"No," I mumbled.

As I drifted into a merciful state of unconsciousness, I heard him say, "You were calling for your daddy."

I came to in the emergency room, where I was treated for hypothermia. My friends had sustained only cuts and bruises.

"You're all lucky," the highway patrolman said. "Especially you, young lady. Those chains are strung across canals to keep animals and debris from flowing into the lake. I can't believe you knew to grab it when you did, or had the strength to in that freezing water."

"I had help," I muttered.

"You must have had help, Mary," the patrolman said. "You were deathly close to being sucked into the underground siphon that pumps water into the lake. Another ten feet, and we'd never have found your body." He patted my shoulder. "Somebody up there is looking after you."

Not just somebody, I thought. *My Daddy.*

That afternoon in the canal was the last time in my life I've been afraid. Even years later, when our infant daughter had open-heart surgery, I had a faith-filled peace no one could understand. I can feel that, with Dad's help, the hand of God is over me. I need only to reach out and grasp it.

Mary Ann Hagen
As told to LeAnn Thieman

Love Can Last Forever

I can honestly say it was the best of times and the worst of times. I was joyfully expecting my first child at the same time that my once-energetic, zestful mother was losing her battle with a brain tumor.

For ten years, my fiercely independent and courageous mother had fought, but none of the surgeries or treatments had been successful. Still, she never lost her ability to smile. But now, finally, at only fifty-five, she became totally disabled—unable to speak, walk, eat or dress on her own.

As she grew closer and closer to death, my baby grew closer and closer to life inside me. My biggest fear was that their lives would never connect. I grieved not only for the upcoming loss of my mother, but also that she and my baby would never know each other.

My fear seemed well-founded. A few weeks before my due date, Mother lapsed into a deep coma. Her doctors did not hold any hope; they told us her time was up. It was useless to put in a feeding tube, they said; she would never awaken.

We brought Mother home to her own bed in her own house, and we insisted on care to keep her comfortable. As often as I could, I sat beside her and talked to her about the baby moving inside me. I hoped that somehow deep inside, she knew.

On February 3, 1989, at about the same time my labor started, Mother opened her eyes. When they told me this at the hospital, I called her home and asked for the phone to be put to Mom's ear.

"Mom—Mom—listen. The baby is coming! You're going to have a new grandchild. Do you understand?"

"Yes!"

What a wonderful word! The first clear word she'd spoken in months!

When I called again an hour later, the nurse at her house told me the impossible: Mom was sitting up, her oxygen tubes removed. She was smiling.

"Mom, it's a boy! You have a new grandson!"

"Yes! Yes! I know!"

Four words. Four beautiful words.

By the time I brought Jacob home, Mom was sitting in her chair, dressed and ready to welcome him. Tears of joy blocked my vision as I laid my son in her arms and she clucked at him. They stared at each other.

They knew.

For two more weeks, Mother clucked, smiled and held Jacob. For two weeks she spoke to my father, her children and grandchildren in complete sentences. For two miracle weeks, she gave us joy.

Then she quietly slipped back into a coma and, after visits from all her children, was finally free of the pain and confines of a body that no longer did her will.

Memories of my son's birth will always be bittersweet for me, but it was at this time that I learned an important truth about living. For while both joy and sorrow are fleeting, and often intertwined, love has the power to overcome both. And love can last forever.

Deb Plouse Fulton

Highway Hero

A miracle cannot prove what is impossible; it is useful only to confirm what is possible . . .

Maimonides

During my third year as a speaker, giving seminars all over the country, I was driving into Wheeling, West Virginia, to teach a class on self-esteem to 150 women.

My background includes being raised by a mother and grandmother who took great pains to teach me that families take care of one another no matter what. I knew I could always count on them when I was in trouble, and they knew they could do the same.

I was driving faster than I should have been because I desperately wanted to make it to Wheeling before the severe rain that had been predicted began to fall.

As I saw the sign telling me Wheeling was eight miles away, I speeded up even a bit more, even though a few raindrops had just begun to fall.

With no warning, I heard a boom—not too loud, but loud enough to know it wasn't a good sound. When I turned off the radio to further evaluate the sound, it became clear I had a tire problem: probably a flat. I slowed down, knowing from high school driver's education not to brake hard, but knowing still that I needed to get off the road for my safety.

On the side of the road, I looked around, saw nothing but rugged hills, a six-lane highway and very fast traffic. I locked the door, to be safe, and tried to figure out what to do. I did not have a cellular phone, as they were not that common many years ago.

Every story I had ever heard about women having bad experiences on the side of the road in strange cities ran through my mind like a movie reel, and I tried to decide if I would be safer staying with the car or walking to the next exit. It was beginning to get dark, and I truly was becoming afraid.

My grandmother taught me as a very little girl that things work out if you keep your head about you, and I was trying very hard to do just that.

At that very moment, a large semi passed very fast on my left, causing my car to shudder, and I saw that the directional light was on, indicating he was pulling over in front of me. I could hear his brakes squeal, as he was braking fast and hard.

I again thought, *Am I safer or in more danger?* I could see the truck as it slowly backed up on the shoulder of the road and decided that to be very safe, I would take a precaution I had seen in a movie. I took out a pad in my briefcase and wrote down the name of the trucking company and the Ohio license number, as they both were visible from my car. I put the pad with this information under the driver's seat just in case!

Even though it was now raining quite hard, the driver came running back from the truck to my car and said through my window that I had opened only three inches, that he had seen the tire blow and would be glad to change it. He asked for the car keys to get into the trunk; and although I knew I was about to lose all my safety precautions, it seemed to be my best choice. I gave him the keys. He changed the tire and gave me back the keys. I asked him through the three-inch opening in the window if I could pay him for his kindness. He said, "We drivers in Ohio believe in taking care of women in trouble on the highway."

I then asked him for the name of his boss so I could send him or her a letter relaying how wonderful he had been. He laughed a very odd laugh and gave me the name of his boss, a woman, and his card, which had the name of the trucking company, the address and the phone number. I thanked him again, and the now soaking-wet man ran back to the truck. Gratefully, I went on to Wheeling to present my seminar.

Upon returning to Florida, I had a T-shirt made for this man that showed an angel in a truck with the words printed across the picture, "Highway Hero," and sent it to the address on the card.

It came back, addressee unknown.

I called the number on the card and got a recording saying no such number existed. I called the city newspaper for that town, asked for the editor, explained the dilemma and asked that a letter to the editor be placed in the paper thanking the driver. The editor, who had lived there all his life, said there was no such company in that city. He further investigated and called me back and said there was no such business registered in Ohio.

The editor went one step further. He called the state motor vehicle bureau to ask about the license and was told no such plate had ever been issued.

The upshot is that this man, his truck and the company never existed, the "rescue" never happened and I must have been dreaming.

But I know I wasn't.

Carol A. Price-Lopata

Plenty of Sunsets

My heart sank when I saw the yellow Volkswagen bug up ahead on the side of the road. The hood was raised, and a young man was gazing down at the engine with an air of hopelessness. Sure enough, my friend, Michael, stepped on the brake and said, "Looks like someone's in trouble."

I sighed with resignation. In our three months of traveling around the United States together, I had learned that Michael would never pass up an opportunity to help someone. Regardless of our personal situation (which, admittedly, was pretty carefree), he leapt at any chance to rescue stranded motorists, pick up hitchhikers and lend a hand wherever he could.

And there were plenty of opportunities to help. This was 1974, and we were part of the masses of young Americans who had taken to the highways, either hitchhiking or driving cars so old they ran on a hope and a prayer. One day in Utah, we picked up so many hitchhikers that there was standing room only in our Chevy van. Once we spent two days in Missoula, Montana, because a young family we picked up had no place to go. Michael knew someone who knew someone in Missoula, and before we left, "our" family had a place to stay and a new start on life.

I loved Michael's generosity and kindness, but I thought he overdid it just a tad. "There are other people driving on these roads," I'd point out. "Can't we *ever* leave somebody for someone else to help?" He'd listen to me. He'd smile at me. He'd stop for the next hitchhiker.

Sometimes I got angry when he put strangers' needs above my own. "But I wanted to see the sun set on the Pacific," I once wailed as we pulled off the road and stopped behind a steaming vehicle. He laughed. "There are plenty of sunsets ahead for you."

But today was different. It was the end of our trip, and we were actually in a bit of a hurry. We had left Florida that morning with the goal of getting home to Massachusetts for Christmas, and Christmas was just two days away. Not only that, but our beloved van was on its last legs. We had already stopped once that morning for emergency repairs.

That had been enough adventure for one day, I thought. I replayed the scene in my head. Michael had seen the billowing steam and pulled over to the side of the road. He diagnosed the problem at a glance, he grabbed a can and headed down into the roadside ditch. I grabbed a cup and climbed down into the ditch after him. We filled the radiator with swamp water and headed off again, thinking we were pretty smart. But suddenly, just a few yards down the road, we started shrieking and slapping our ankles. Michael swerved to the side of the road and we spilled out of the car. Ants! Tiny ants swarmed on our calves and ankles, biting us hard. We kicked off our shoes and socks and howled and slapped till the last little ant was dead. As we climbed back in, I said a heartfelt prayer that we wouldn't have to go down into any more Florida ditches.

Now, as we pulled to a stop behind the VW, I made one last appeal. "Michael, please," I begged, "can't we *please* just get ourselves and this poor old van home in time for Christmas?" As he hopped out to check out the problem, he said, "We'll get there, honey. Don't worry."

A minute later he was back with the young man in tow. "We need to get some help. We'll get off at the exit right up ahead."

When we pulled into a gas station at the foot of the exit, I waited in the car, sulking just a little at my defeat. Suddenly, I felt very strange all over my body. I looked at my hands and saw huge welts bloom at my wrists. I looked in the rear view mirror and gasped at the gray and red blotches swelling on my face. Hives! I felt a choking sensation, and started gasping for air. In a panic, I fumbled with the car door, got it open and staggered toward Michael and the mechanics. "Michael! Michael!" I called in a weak and panic-stricken voice.

Michael turned and his face filled with horror. He ran toward me, calling to the mechanics, "Where's the nearest hospital?"

"That way. Two blocks down on the left."

Michael started driving before we had the doors shut. I gasped and choked and struggled to breathe while he yelled, "Hang on, honey, just hang on! Just hang on."

He raced down the street and swerved to a stop at the entrance of the hospital. I ran into the lobby and fell to the floor. I couldn't catch my breath to call for help, but nurses came running and lifted me onto a gurney.

Within seconds, a gentle doctor with a gray beard was asking me questions. I choked out, "There were ants . . . side of the road," and pointed to my ankles. He filled a huge hypodermic and said, "Just relax. You're going to be all right. You've had such a bad allergic reaction you've got hives on the inside of your lungs."

The shot he gave me started to work. Breathing comfortably again, I asked, "Would I have died?"

"You probably had about five more minutes," he said.

Thirty minutes later, Michael and I walked out of the hospital and climbed back into the van. We got back onto the highway, and the first thing we saw was a sign: "Next exit forty miles." I looked at Michael and burst into tears. If we hadn't stopped for that VW and then taken the next exit, I would have died. I would have been forty miles from help and gasping for air.

Two nights later, on Christmas Eve, we pulled into my parents' driveway. Through the snow-drifted windows, I saw my family in the warmly lit living room, laughing and joking as they decorated the tree. Before we went in, I hugged Michael and thanked him again, one more time, for everything. He hugged me back and laughed, "Didn't I tell you you'd see plenty of sunsets?"

Cindy Jevne Buck

Mom, Can You Pull Some Strings?

"Mom, you can't die. I'm a late bloomer," I pleaded at my mother's bedside, as she lay dying of pancreatic/liver cancer. This couldn't be happening! My beautiful, vibrant, effervescent, fifty-nine-year-old mother couldn't be sick! It was all so unreal. Just two months ago she was fine, and yet now here she was, days from death.

"Mom, you have to meet my future husband and kids. You're not done."

"Oh, Carol, I would have loved that," she said, wanly.

"Okay, Mom. If you're not going to meet him, you have to send him to me! Will you pull some strings for me up there?" I asked, trying to make her feel better.

"Yeah, Mom, you're on loser patrol. Carol needs help," my older sister, Linda, chimed in. We'd both moved home to nurse Mom and were with her night and day. Linda was right. I did need help. I'd dated a string of unavailable men. I'd been broken-hearted several times.

"Oh, my God. I don't want that job! I'm supposed to be resting up there," Mom exclaimed, knowing all too well how difficult the subject of "Mr. Right" was for me.

"Well, in that case, Mom, while you're at it, do you

think you could get me a book deal?" asked Linda only half-joking. She'd been working on a book for three years and had a handful of rejection slips from numerous publishers.

"Gee, you two! I'll see what I can do," she said, smiling weakly.

A few days later, Mom passed away peacefully, the two of us praying by her side, our weeping father at the foot of the bed.

At her memorial service, Linda and I recounted for the over 300 attendees what a giving, selfless, loving mother she was.

I told the story of the first time she met the most significant boyfriend in my turbulent past, Bill. Bill was a professional harmonica player. On this first meeting, we went to brunch with my parents for Easter. Bill was my first real boyfriend after high school—the first relationship I'd had in six years. My parents were understandably excited to be meeting him. I was very nervous and hopeful that all would go well. Much to my horror, my father was barraging Bill with a series of annoying questions before we'd even ordered. "When was the harmonica invented? . . . What keys do they come in? . . . How many can you play?" And on and on. I wanted to melt underneath my chair! I looked desperately to my mother for help. Noticing my frantic eyes, she chimed in, "So, Bill, how long have you two been seeing each other?"

This was helping?!

"Uh, about six months," Bill replied.

"Gee," said Mom, leaning forward and grinning widely, "Any thoughts of this getting serious?" I wanted to die.

"Not until this very moment," Bill responded dryly.

In spite of it all, Bill and I went on to date for three years. He treated me like a queen and I grew to love him more every day. He felt ready to get married. I did not. We consequently broke up. I felt certain a world of wonderful men was waiting for me with open arms. I was wrong. With every new failed relationship, I'd weep to Linda, "Bill was so much better for me." He, on the other hand, was in a committed relationship almost immediately after we broke up. I was devastated!

Bill and his new love moved 1,000 miles away to New Mexico after a year. I hoped this would make things easier. As fate would have it, Linda called one day to inform me that she and her family had discovered an incredible land opportunity through Bill and were moving to New Mexico as well, with Bill and his girlfriend right next door. They would never be out of my life.

For Christmas, three months after Mom's death, my father and I went to see Linda and her family. I was very depressed without Mom.

We went to a big Christmas dinner. Bill was there. His girlfriend was away working for a few months. For the first time in the four years since we'd broken up, I felt very comfortable—as if he were an old friend. I was finally over it.

Two nights later, I was still really missing Mom. I decided to talk to her—something I had not yet done since she had died. I was staying by myself in a trailer a few minutes from Linda's. I lit a candle and said, "Mom, I miss you. Come be with me." The whole trailer immediately filled with brilliant white light. It was like nothing I had ever seen before. I could see it just as brightly with my eyes closed. "Mom, is that you?" I asked. The light flickered in response. She had come! Very at peace, I went to sleep, the light of my mother's essence encircling me.

Later that week, I had dinner with Bill. He confessed that he was still in love with me and that he couldn't get me out of his mind.

"How long have you been feeling this way?" I asked, incredulous.

"It's been especially intense since I saw you after your mother died. One look, and I knew we'd be together," he explained. I was completely in shock. "I've been talking to your mother about this," he said sweetly. "And you remember that first dinner I had with your mother when she asked if we were getting serious?" he said with a twinkle. "I think that meant she approves."

We were married nine months later.

Linda sold her book to a very reputable, successful publishing company the month before our nuptials.

I sure hope Mom can get that rest now.

Carol Allen

Never, Never Give Up

It was a very exciting day for us—the championship Little League game of the season. Two teams would be battling it out one more time for the championship. We were the only team all season to beat this "Paint Shop" team, and they were determined to win tonight's game.

We were a baseball family. Ben, my husband, had coached the Little League team for the past two years, but he had lost his battle to cancer two months earlier. Dying at the age of forty-three after a courageous struggle, he had left me and our two children, Jared, ten, and Lara, six.

He had coached while undergoing massive doses of chemotherapy and many stays in the hospital, along with daily trips to the hospital for tests. Despite being tired, worried and worn down, he had continued to coach.

How he delighted in Jared's accomplishments playing baseball, and how proud he would have been today of this team and Jared, the team leader and starting pitcher.

Ben was an English teacher by profession and had enjoyed coaching soccer and baseball for years. He taught the teams how to play the game and about good sportsmanship, fair play and physical fitness. He also taught his family and a caring community how to fight a terrible disease with faith, hope, courage and dignity. He gave us all the courage to hope when all hope was lost.

An avid reader, Ben jotted down quotes on index cards and left them here or there around the house. One quote he loved was by Winston Churchill during World War II: "Never, never, never, never give up." It seemed so appropriate for Ben, as those were the words he lived by, fighting this disease for one-and-a-half years, up to his very last breath. Upon his death, we had those words inscribed on his tombstone. Those special words became a message to my children and me upon every visit to his grave. They were not something to be shared—they were just for us. Our secret message to each other from Dad.

The game was close, and Jared felt the pressure.

Because parents, family and friends on both teams had helped care for our children at a moment's notice during our nightmare and had felt much anguish upon Ben's death, every person at that field missed Ben that evening.

One enthusiastic father, whose son was new to the team, and who had not known our family circumstances over the past year, came to the game with twenty-five paper cups on which he had written different baseball expressions: "Get a base hit," "Catch that fly ball," "Pop-Up," "Bunt." What fun it would be for each player to read a message on his cup after quenching his thirst.

The score was close; it was a nerve-wracking game. In the fourth inning, Jared pulled a cup out randomly for his drink of water. Suddenly he ran from the bench over to me with the cup. Written on his cup were the words, "Never, never give up." The news spread fast. Ben was there, even if in spirit only. Needless to say, we won the game, and the cup now sits on a shelf next to Ben's picture to greet anyone who walks in our back door.

Diane Novinski

The Baby Blanket

A coincidence is a small miracle where God chose to remain anonymous . . .

Heidi Quade

It was a spring Saturday, and though many activities clamored for my attention, I had chosen this time to sit and crochet, an activity I enjoyed but had once thought impossible.

Most of the time I don't mind being a "lefty"—I'm quite proud of it, actually. But I admit, it did cause me a few problems three years ago, when I wanted to help out with a project at church.

We were invited to crochet baby blankets, which would be donated to a local Crisis Pregnancy Center at Christmas. I wanted to participate but I knew nothing about how to crochet, and my left-handedness didn't help. I had trouble "thinking backwards."

I suppose where there is a will, there is a way, because a few of the ladies got together and taught me one stitch. That's all I needed. I learned that granny stitch, and before long I had a blanket made. I was so proud of my little accomplishment and it seemed, inexplicably, so important, that I made quite a few more that same year. I even included in each blanket, as a note of encouragement, a poem I had written that read:

> Little girls are sweet in their ruffles all pink.
> Little boys in overalls look divine.
> But no matter which one that the Lord gives to you,
> A better "Mom" he never could find.

All of a sudden, my thoughts were interrupted by the ringing of my telephone. I hurried to answer it, and to my surprise and delight, on the other end of the line was Karen Sharp, who had been one of my very best friends ever since elementary school. Karen, her husband, Jim, and their daughter, Kim, had moved away a few years ago. She was calling to say that she was in town for a couple of days and would like to come by. I was thrilled to hear her voice.

At last the doorbell rang. As I flung open the door, we both screamed, as if back in junior high. We hugged each other. Then questions began to fly. Finally, I guided Karen into the kitchen, where I poured a cool glass of tea for both of us and the conversation slowed.

To my delight, Karen seemed to be calm, rested and, most of all, self-assured, which were a few qualities that she had seemed to lose during the last few months before they moved away. I wondered what had caused the positive change.

As we talked and reminisced, Karen began to explain to me the true reasons for her family's move a few years ago. The original reason they had given me was that Jim had a job offer in another city, which they could not afford to pass up. Even though it was Kim's senior year in high school, they still felt it necessary to make the move. Apparently, that had not been the biggest reason.

Karen reached into her purse and pulled out a photograph. When she handed it to me, I saw it was a beautiful little girl—maybe about two or three years old.

"This is my granddaughter, Kayla," Karen said.

I couldn't believe my ears. "You're a *grandmother?*" I asked. "I don't understand."

"You see," Karen went on, "Kim was a few months pregnant when we moved away. We had just found out, and Kim was having a really rough time dealing with it—she even talked about suicide. We were frantic. So we decided to move away, hoping that she would adjust more easily. When we finally settled in our new home, we hoped that Kim's outlook would begin to improve, but she became more and more depressed. No matter what we said, she felt worthless and like a failure. Then we found a woman named Mrs. Barber, a wonderful pregnancy counselor. She got Kim through some very tough times.

"As the time for delivery came closer, Kim still had not entirely made up her mind about whether to keep the baby or not. Her father and I prayed that she would. We felt prepared to give the baby a loving home—it was, after all, our first grandchild!

"Finally, the day came, and Kim had a six-pound, six-ounce baby girl. Mrs. Barber came to visit her in the hospital. She hugged Kim and told her how proud she was of her. Then she gave Kim a pastel-colored package containing a hand-crocheted baby blanket inside."

At this point, I felt a huge lump come into my throat, and I felt rather limp all over, but I tried not to show my feelings and kept listening to Karen's story.

Karen must have noticed the look on my face. She asked if I was all right. I assured her I was fine and asked her to please continue.

"As I said," she went on, "there was a baby blanket and a little personal note, something about little girls and their ruffles, little boys and their overalls, and a word of encouragement about becoming a new mom.

"We asked who made the blanket, and Mrs. Barber explained that some of the pregnancy centers have people who donate these blankets to new mothers and their babies. Her center was given the surplus from one of the other centers in the state, and she was glad to have one for Kim.

"Kim was so moved by the fact that a total stranger had thought enough to put this much time and effort into a blanket for her baby. She said it made her feel warm all over. She later told her dad and me that the little poem gave her a boost of confidence and helped her to make up her mind to keep little Kayla."

Karen's story had an even happier ending: A year later, Kim was married to a young man who loves both her and Kayla with all his heart. Karen grinned as she told me, then sobered. "My only regret is that I did not feel close enough to our friends here to have been able to lean on you all for support and comfort, instead of turning away.

"We are so thankful for so many things—especially the way everything turned out; but I think the one thing that we are the most thankful for is that kind person who made that little baby blanket for our daughter and her baby. I just wish I could give her a big hug and tell her how much she is loved and appreciated by our family."

I looked again at the photo of the sweet child in my hands. Then I leaned over to Karen and gave her a big hug.

Winona Smith

10

ACROSS THE GENERATIONS

*Life is no brief candle to me. It is a sort of
splendid torch which I have got hold of for
the moment, and I want to make it burn as
brightly as possible before handing it on
to future generations.*

George Bernard Shaw

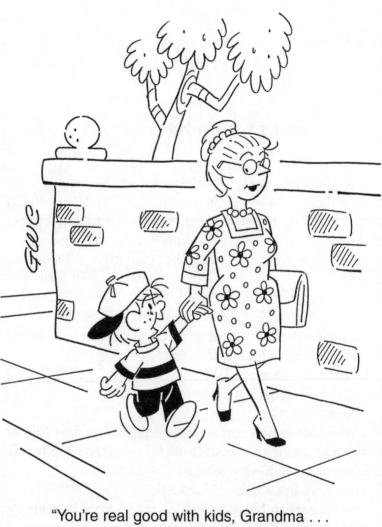

"You're real good with kids, Grandma . . .
you ought to have some of your own."

Reprinted by permission of George Crenshaw.

Stories on a Headboard

The bed was about forty-five years old when Mom passed it along to me a few months after my father died. I decided to strip the wood and refinish it for my daughter Melanie. The headboard was full of scratches.

Just before starting to take the paint off, I noticed that one of the scratches was a date: September 18, 1946, the day my parents were married. Then it struck me—this was the first bed they had as husband and wife!

Right above their wedding date was another name and date: "Elizabeth, October 22, 1947."

I called my mother. "Who is Elizabeth," I asked, "and what does October 22, 1947, mean?"

"She's your sister."

I knew Mom had lost a baby, but I never saw this as anything more than a misfortune for my parents. After all, they went on to have five more children.

"You gave her a name?" I asked.

"Yes. Elizabeth has been watching us from heaven for forty-five years. She's as much a part of me as any of you."

"Mom, there are a lot of dates and names I don't recognize on the headboard."

"June 8, 1959?" Mom asked.

"Yes. It says 'Sam.'"

"Sam was a black man who worked for your father at the plant. Your father was fair with everyone, treating those under him with equal respect, no matter what their race or religion. But there was a lot of racial tension at that time. There was also a union strike and a lot of trouble.

"One night, some strikers surrounded your dad before he got to his car. Sam showed up with several friends, and the crowd dispersed. No one was hurt. The strike eventually ended, but your dad never forgot Sam. He said Sam was an answer to his prayer."

"Mom, there are other dates on the headboard. May I come over and talk to you about them?" I sensed the headboard was full of stories. I couldn't just strip and sand them away.

Over lunch, Mom told me about January 14, 1951, the day she lost her purse at a department store. Three days later, the purse arrived in the mail. A letter from a woman named Amy said: "I took five dollars from your wallet to mail the purse to you. I hope you will understand." There was no return address, so Mom couldn't thank her, and there was nothing missing except the five dollars.

Then there was George. On December 15, 1967, George shot a rattlesnake poised to strike my brother Dominick. On September 18, 1971, my parents celebrated their silver wedding anniversary and renewed their vows.

I learned about a nurse named Janet who stayed by my mother and prayed with her after my sister Patricia's near-fatal fall from a swing. There was a stranger who broke up the attempted mugging of my father but left without giving his name.

"Who is Ralph?" I asked.

"On February 18, 1966, Ralph saved your brother's life

in Da Nang. Ralph was killed two years later on his second tour of duty."

My brother never spoke about the Vietnam War. The memories were deeply buried. My nephew's name is Ralph. Now I knew why.

"I almost stripped away these remarkable stories," I said. "How could you give this headboard to me?"

"Your dad and I carved our first date on the headboard the night we married. From then on, it was a diary of our life together. When Dad died, our life together was over. But the memories never die."

When I told my husband about the headboard, he said, "There's room for a lot more stories."

We moved the bed with the story-book headboard into our room. My husband and I have already carved in three dates and names. Someday, we'll tell Melanie the stories from her grandparents' lives and the stories from her parents' lives. And someday, the bed will pass on to her.

Elaine Pondant

Mother's Hands

Love is patient, love is kind. It does not envy, it does not boast, it is not proud. It is not rude, it is not self-seeking, it is not easily angered, it keeps no record of wrongs....

1 Cor. 13:4-5

Night after night, she came to tuck me in, even long after my childhood years. Following her longstanding custom, she'd lean down and push my long hair out of the way, then kiss my forehead.

I don't remember when it first started annoying me—her hands pushing my hair that way. But it did annoy me, for they felt work-worn and rough against my young skin. Finally, one night, I lashed out at her: "Don't *do* that any-more—your hands are too rough!" She didn't say anything in reply. But never again did my mother close out my day with that familiar expression of her love. Lying awake long afterward, my words haunted me. But pride stifled my conscience, and I didn't tell her I was sorry.

Time after time, with the passing years, my thoughts returned to that night. By then I missed my mother's hands, missed her goodnight kiss upon my forehead. Sometimes the incident seemed very close, sometimes far away. But always it lurked, hauntingly, in the back of my mind.

Well, the years have passed, and I'm not a little girl anymore. Mom is in her mid-seventies, and those hands I once thought to be so rough are still doing things for me and my family. She's been our doctor, reaching into a medicine cabinet for the remedy to calm a young girl's stomach or soothe a boy's scraped knee. She cooks the best fried chicken in the world . . . gets stains out of blue jeans like I never could . . . and still insists on dishing out ice cream at any hour of the day or night.

Through the years, my mother's hands have put in countless hours of toil, and most of hers were before perma-pressed fabrics and automatic washers!

Now, my own children are grown and gone. Mom no longer has Dad, and on special occasions, I find myself drawn next door to spend the night with her. So it was that late one Thanksgiving Eve, as I drifted into sleep in the bedroom of my youth, a familiar hand hesitantly stole across my face to brush the hair from my forehead. Then a kiss, ever so gently, touched my brow.

In my memory, for the thousandth time, I recalled the night my surly young voice complained: "Don't *do* that anymore—your hands are too rough!" I reacted involuntarily. Catching Mom's hand in mine, I blurted out how sorry I was for that night. I thought she'd remember, as I did. But Mom didn't know what I was talking about. She had forgotten—and forgiven—long ago.

That night, I fell asleep with a new appreciation for my gentle mother and her caring hands. And the guilt I had carried around for so long was nowhere to be found.

Louisa Godissart McQuillen

Every Woman Needs a Champion

Every child needs a champion—a person who cherishes her and supports her every step of the way. My champion was Lillian, a woman my mother's age, but a close friend of my grandmother's.

My earliest memory of Lillian occurred when I was three. Her only daughter and my eldest sister, both tyrannical six-year-olds, refused to let me climb her apple tree. They called me a big baby—a crushing insult to one so recently out of diapers. Lillian strode over, scooped me off the ground and plunked me down on the lowest branch of the tree, soothing me by crooning to me, "Ca-Coo," a pet name she had given me before my first birthday. Then she brought me a cookie—a Viennese crescent she got from the best bakery in New York—and initiated the first of a lifetime of serious talks.

"Come, sit down, Ca-Coo," she would say. "Tell me about yourself." Although busy with her own friends and work, Lillian took the time to listen to the trials of a not-so-eager kindergartner, a defiant tomboy, an awkward adolescent and a rebellious college student. While my own parents were practically pulling out their hair, Lillian never criticized. She never stopped calling me Ca-Coo, and she never stopped offering Viennese crescent cookies from the best bakery in New York.

Lillian took an interest in my dating life. As I paraded a stream of boyfriends through her door, she always served my favorite cookies and made my suitors feel welcome. When the inevitable break-ups occurred, Lillian helped pick up the shattered pieces, and never said, "I thought he was a louse to begin with." When I finally settled down with the man who eventually became my husband, Lillian prepared a five-course dinner for just the three of us. She called me Ca-Coo and for dessert served Viennese crescent cookies from the best bakery in New York.

I married my husband while he was in graduate school, and the only work I could find was as a part-time teacher in a private school. My meager salary didn't stretch far and I felt poverty-stricken. Lillian called one day and said, "Ca-Coo, just listen and don't say anything. I have five-hundred dollars for you sitting in my bank account. If you need money for any reason, just call and I'll send it to you. No questions asked." Then she hung up.

Suddenly, I felt rich. I had a buffer. I never used it. My husband finished school, got a good-paying job, and we started a family. Lillian oohed and ahhed over our children. After the birth of each, she reminded me of the emergency fund she still held for me. I was touched. Hard times had fallen on Lillian—her husband had died. She was short on cash, but always long on love. But I knew that if I ever called, the five-hundred dollars would be mine.

I did call Lillian—lots of times over the years. The conversations always started the same way.

"Hi, Lillian? This is Carole."

"Who?"

I knew she knew who I was, but I played along. "Lillian, it's me, Ca-Coo."

"Ca-Coo, darling!" she responded with joy. "Tell me how you're doing."

I would smile. She would never let me grow up.

When I was in my late twenties, I told Lillian I wanted to become a writer. She responded enthusiastically and became my greatest cheerleader. When my books were published, she'd buy them in bulk and mail them to me to autograph. She'd then dispatch them to her friends and relatives. It didn't matter to her that I wrote children's books and that the recipients were full-grown.

When I was thirty-three, I injured my back and could not leave my bed for seven months. Throughout this ordeal, Lillian called me weekly to give me pep talks. I had little new to say. Our relationship gradually changed. Lillian opened up to me, and I became her confidante. Finally, I felt I was able to give back some of the support she had given me.

When I recovered, I brought my children to visit her. Time had not robbed her of her good looks and ability to dress meticulously. She still called me Ca-Coo and served my children Viennese crescent cookies from the best bakery in New York.

A couple of years passed, and I decided to surprise Lillian by dedicating a new book to her. The inscription read, "To Lillian, for always being there."

In January, I visited Lillian for a weekend. She didn't look good. She hadn't been eating right. She yelled at me for growing up. Everything I did or said displeased her, and I left depressed. I called her a few weeks later. She had company and could not talk. She said she'd call back but never did.

I came down with mononucleosis and pneumonia. It had nothing to do with Lillian. I was so busy with my family, my writing and my friends that I neglected myself. Now I had to spend two months regaining my health. I'd think about Lillian but didn't have the energy to call.

Finally I was well again, and scurried about trying to catch up on all the things I couldn't do while ill. I called Lillian's number, but no one answered. For several weeks I tried without success, finally deciding she was probably out of town visiting her daughter. Then in June, my grandmother took me aside.

"Lillian has metastasized breast cancer," she told me. "She is dying. You weren't told sooner because we feared you would have a mono relapse."

I rushed to see Lillian. Walking into the hospital room, I instantly realized I was in the wrong place. Huddled in a wheelchair was an old, balding, emaciated woman. As I was about to apologize for disturbing her, the woman began to speak in a weak, cracking voice.

"Ca-Coo!" she said. "I'm so glad you came. Sit down and tell me about yourself."

We talked for an hour. She told me that soon she would no longer be. I told her that I knew—and that I would miss her. I promised never to forget her.

Three weeks later, my champion was dead. After her funeral, I returned to her apartment with family and friends. My favorite Viennese crescent cookies were set out, but I couldn't eat one. I felt destitute. My buffer was gone. There was no one left to call me Ca-Coo.

Another year passed, and the pain of Lillian's death lost its raw edge. One summer morning, my doorbell rang. Standing by the front door was Laura, the three-year-old daughter of a friend.

"Come sit down, Munchkin," I said. "Tell me all about yourself."

Laura dashed to the couch and plopped herself down. And she waited impatiently while I opened a box of Viennese crescent cookies from the best bakery in town.

Carole Garbuny Vogel

The Trellis

Why is this so hard, I wonder. All I have to do is tack together a few sticks of wood and daub them with white paint, but I feel as if I'm making a cross for my own execution. Already I've gone through a tablet full of designs and a forest of pine lath. I want this to be right.

"I'd like a white trellis," was your modest request. "Something for a background at my wedding. Sarah Parkes will cover it with ivy. It will be beautiful, Daddy, a symbol of life."

I was glad you asked me to make the trellis because I wanted to have a part in the wedding. Seems like men are mostly in the way at such occasions—like chess pieces standing around, waiting to be "positioned." The groom himself would never be missed if he didn't show. They would just stand a cardboard cutout in his place and no one would be the wiser.

Weddings are of women, by women and for women. But with this trellis, I can have a part of the action.

If I can ever get it made.

I've made far more difficult things for you, like that colonial cradle for your doll, and that two-story dollhouse with handmade furnishings. And your desk, with all the drawers.

But this trellis!

Kneeling on the patio, I carefully weave the pine slats into a crosshatch, and a design slowly emerges. As I work, I ponder the way your life has woven itself into mine, and I wonder what I will be like without Natalie around the house.

Can we unweave twenty-one years of sharing? Can a father give away his daughter without coming a little unraveled himself?

It's not that I don't want you to marry. I do. When your dreams come true, so do mine. Matt is such a good choice. A gentle, handsome man, as devoted to you as your parents. "Nat and Matt" sounds right, like a little poem.

I can hardly see to drive these tiny nails. Allergies, probably. Or maybe it's the cool April breeze that keeps fogging my eyes. Or the smart scent of pine wood.

They will stand this trellis up on the stage at church. My job is to take you by the arm and gently lead you down the aisle to the trellis. Another man will help you up the next step of life. I'll sit there stoically with your mother, watching you embrace someone new. Your sister will sing your favorite songs. Your grandfathers will perform the ceremony. And God will come down to bless the union. Your mother has it all organized.

All I have to do is finish this simple trellis.

When the wedding is over, they will fold this ivy arbor and shove it into a dark storage room, where it will be forever forgotten. But memories of my little girl will vine themselves through the arbor of my heart for the rest of my years.

I stand the trellis up against the garage and slather it with bride-white paint—this fragrant veneer that covers the old, rugged tree with beauty and promise.

Painted, the trellis looks like two alabaster gates. Gates

that lead to a future I may never see, if you move far away. Out there on the long road of daily living, who knows what will happen? There will be long days filled with sweet monotony. Bright moments of joy. And tedious hours of sorrow. I wish for you the full spectrum of life.

I rub the syrupy paint from my fingers with a rag that used to be your favorite T-shirt. Then I stand back to appraise my work.

Without the ivy it seems so empty and lonely.

It is, after all, just a simple trellis.

And it is finished.

But it's the hardest thing I've ever made.

Daniel Schantz

A Final Letter to a Father

*Come death, if you will: you cannot divide us;
you can only unite us . . .*

Franz Grillparger

Dear Dad,

A year has passed since your children placed a collection of greeting cards on the kitchen table, hoping against hope that you would awaken in the morning to read them. But you slipped away in the darkness of the night, determined, I'm sure, to spare us the additional anguish of losing you on Father's Day.

This year there will be no cards at all. Just this, my final letter to you.

For quite some time after your death, I kept reaching into my mailbox expecting to hear from you. From the time I moved away from home years ago, your letters were a constant reassurance in my unpredictable life. Yours were funny, newsy missives pounded out regularly on your clunker of a typewriter: Movies to see and to avoid. The latest scandals at the university. Your travels around the globe with Mom. Jay's graduation from law school and his engagement to Debra—on my birthday! Mitch's adventures in Hollywood. Births, deaths and divorces.

Sometimes they contained money I hadn't asked for; somehow you knew.

I kept every letter you wrote to me, thinking that when I was a very old woman, I would dust off the boxes and unwrap each one like a precious present . . . every typewritten sheet chronicling a piece of our family's life and the world as it evolved year after year. How could I have known I'd be reaching into those boxes so soon?

December 10, 1987

You speak of the year's end with the exuberance that has always marked your letters. Your students, suffering from predictable "bouts of hysteria and anxiety," are preparing for finals. Holiday invitations are rolling in, and cousins are coming to town to help you ring in the New Year. You wish Barry and me luck as we voyage cross-country to Minnesota, suggesting that we start practicing how to keep warm. "Body heat," you suggest wryly, "is a good first step."

January 12, 1988

You don't mention the cancer, diagnosed three days before Christmas, until the fourth paragraph. First you ask about life in Siberia . . . uh . . . Minnesota, and assure me that I am the best writer of my generation. Of course. Finally, you tell me that your oncologist has suggested an experimental treatment program in Arizona. "What the hell?" you say. "I'll try it." In the meantime you insist that life will go on normally. You promise me you'll live to 100.

January 22, 1988

I learn that you had your hair cut, ran into Connie, brunched with friends, are struggling with your income taxes and have decided to cancel a trip to New York, "because the weather is so unpredictable this time of year." Before closing, you mention that the medication is giving you flu-like symptoms, and you apologize for making so many errors with the typewriter. I hadn't noticed. It's been a rough go, you finally admit, but you're hanging in there. "Wrap up warmly," you lovingly close, "and say your prayers for me."

March 14, 1988

The tidbits of daily life have been relegated to the final paragraphs. You begin by telling me how grateful you are for every day and how appreciative you have become of the natural things in life. You continue to set goals and feel hopeful. You're looking forward to early retirement. You joke about your weight loss, describing yourself as a "prune face," and assure me that by the time Barry and I arrive at the end of the month, you will have put on some pounds. I send ahead a six-pack of a high-calorie, liquid-protein drink in coffee, your favorite flavor. I am beginning to feel helpless.

April 7, 1988

You and Mom are looking forward to visiting us in Minneapolis. You thank me for understanding that you'd be more comfortable in a hotel. You've begun to clean out your massive collection of office files in anticipation of retirement, although it's a major project that you plan to work on all summer. All summer, you say, and I rejoice. How dramatically my perspective has changed. Just three months ago, I feared you wouldn't be able to keep your promise of living to 100. Today I pray that you'll be here to see the leaves change from green to gold in September.

I set down your letter, and my mind is flooded
with memories. My father, whose sweet voice

sang me to sleep as a child, who accompanied me on my 5 a.m. paper route without a single grumble, taught me French, coached me through adolescence and addressed all 200 invitations to my wedding ... what would my world be like without you in it?

May 23, 1988

Your weakening hand has drawn my name and address on the envelope, using liquid paper to cover up your mistakes. I slowly open the flap and stare blankly at words running together and misspellings that you—always a stickler for correct grammar—have tried diligently to correct. "This typewriter is slowly breaking down," you explain. "We really need to think about buying a word processor." For one precious moment, I feel euphoric: You are going to get well! You are going to buy a word processor! But your closing words jerk me back to reality. "Stay well, happy and no sad songs for me," you write. "And when you think of me, smile."

A week later, I realize that there will never be another letter. I pick up the telephone and hear your voice, asking me to come home.

A year has passed since your death on Father's Day eve, June 18, 1988. At the time, I was certain I'd never again be able to walk past the Father's Day cards in the grocery store without falling apart. But a week ago, I found myself browsing through hundreds of them, the silly, the serious, the sentimental, and I had no trouble buying one. It was for Barry, your devoted son-in-law, who became a father less than two months ago.

And so the cycle continues. Birth, death, then the wonder and magic of birth again. But as my role in life shifts from child to parent, I realize that no one will ever replace you—my father of abundant humor, courage and grace—or your wonderful, although sometimes painful, letters that blanketed me in warmth and documented my world until my twenty-ninth year of life.

Rest peacefully, Dad, and know that when I think of you on this Father's Day, and on every other day, there will be no sad songs. Only smiles.

Your loving daughter,
Gail

Gail Rosenblum

A Penny Saved

Those who love deeply never grow old; they may die of old age, but they die young.

Benjamin Franklin

My mother used to say, "You cost me a pretty penny!" And I did. When both my brother and sister were grown and gone from home, my parents discovered that another baby was on the way. At the age of forty-three, in a small-town hospital in 1937, my mother gave birth—to me. The total bill came to a whopping forty-seven dollars back then. Can you imagine? Forty-seven dollars! A pretty penny indeed!

We were not people of means, but Mother was industrious and creative. "Waste not, want not" was her motto. Many evenings, I fell asleep to the rhythmic thump and whir of her treadle sewing machine. Crisp, polished cottons and sturdy, nubby woolens slid under the needle as she sewed into the quiet hours of the night, copying current styles so that I was well-dressed.

Mother scraped together funds to provide musical training. The house rang with noise—my fingers tripping over the piano keys, my bow grating across violin strings, screeching like a cat with its tail caught under a rocking chair.

Our voices harmonized in favorite songs. We were a barbershop quartet—minus two—when we sang "By the Light of the Silvery Moon," or "In the Good Old Summertime." Sometimes we were the Andrew Sisters singing "The White Cliffs of Dover" and "Till We Meet Again." Oh, and how we loved show hits like "Happy Days Are Here Again" and "Tea for Two."

Mother taught me to tell the truth. She taught me how to shift gears smoothly in our gray 1937 Packard motorcar that we christened "Eunice." She taught me the value of working for the things you want.

Mother was as popular with my friends as she was with me. Each time we entered the kitchen, we were greeted with the aromas of mouth-watering fudge, piping hot potato donuts, juicy gooseberry pie or yeasty homemade bread. Those were welcoming smells. They meant comfort. They meant home.

During my college years in the 1950s, Mother and I maintained our close relationship by correspondence, sharing our thoughts, opinions and experiences. To save money on postage, we developed the unique talent of squeezing lots of words in the tiniest space on a penny postcard. Not an inch was wasted. After all, "A penny saved is a penny earned."

My five children were born during her late seventies, and she visited as frequently as possible. At age eighty-eight, Mother came to live with our family full-time.

We eagerly shuffled our household to accommodate her. She loved going everywhere with me, pushing grocery carts, going to lunch at *her* favorite restaurant, McDonald's. As we drove, she would chant, "One for the money, two for the show, three to get ready, and four to go!"

Those were happy years. When little Matthew wanted attention, he knew just where to go to get it. He nestled next to Grandma's lilac-scented plumpness. She was always good for a cuddle. And she would smooth his hair as she read his favorite book over and over and over again—without saying "Enough!" or leaving out any of the words. Grandma was never in a hurry.

To my twin daughters, Grandma was a soul mate. They paraded their wardrobes, friends and dates before her approving eyes. Grandma always gave her undivided attention.

My teenage boys aired their complaints to her. She knew when to tease, when to sympathize, when to listen. And Grandma always had time to listen.

But as the years slipped away, so did Mother. First it was a cane. Then a walker. Later, no more going up and down stairs. It hurt to see time catching up with her. Sagely, she said, "Poor health is like a bad penny; it's bound to show up sooner or later." Now it was *my* turn to care for *her.*

I carried all her meals upstairs, sat with her in my big bedroom, watching television, ironing, mending, doing my paperwork—keeping her company while she did needlework. We talked. We reminisced. We sang our old favorites, blissfully uncaring that—between the two of us—we *still* couldn't carry a tune in a bucket. I bought yarn, and she crocheted afghans. But one day she put down her crochet hook and never took it up again.

Mother was fading and so was her eyesight. Now it was an older Matthew who climbed the stairs. He nudged Grandma over, squeezed next to her in bed and took *his* turn reading to *her.* And he never left out any of the words.

When I massaged her frail body with lotion or powdered her soft skin, I kissed her velvety back. "You know, *this* spot doesn't look ninety-five years old," I teased.

As she slipped further away, new tasks were necessary. First, it was bathing and bathroom needs, then dressing, and finally, grinding food, spoon-feeding . . . diapering. Our roles changed. I felt that I was now *her* mother, she was *my* child, and we were both enduring to the end.

Six months before her ninety-eighth birthday, Mother peacefully passed away in the comfort of her own little bed, in her own little room . . . in my house. Downstairs in the kitchen, yeast bread was rising, filling the air with the scent of comfort, the scent of home.

As one last act of service, I chose to dress my mother's sweet, aged body—this time for burial. And I felt our roles reverse a second time as once again I became the child, mourning the loss of my mother.

Now, most people don't get to keep their mothers for ninety-seven years. I was blessed to have her, tend her, perhaps even repay her a little for her great sacrifices during my childhood. As I pore over her penny postcards that I've cherished through the years, I can only think: a pretty penny, indeed!

Carita Barlow
As told to Carol McAdoo Rehme

Emma's Bouquets

It was a hot June day when my mother and I crossed the Texas border and made our way to Minden, west of Shreveport, Louisiana. Although it wasn't far to the old George family farm, where my great-grandparents had homesteaded 100 years earlier, I had never been there before.

As we drew closer to the family homestead, through softly rolling hills of longleaf pine, sweet gum and red oak, I thought about what connects us with earlier generations of our family. Is it just a matter of eye color, height or blood type? Or are there other ties that bind us? If my great-grandmother Emma could find her way into the present, would she discover something familiar in my generation?

When my mom and I turned into the George property, we saw before us a real Southern farmhouse—mostly porch with a house attached. Although it was just a simple farmhouse, its front windows were graced with ornately carved dental moldings, and the steps from the porch—flanked by large brick pillars with granite plinths—were a palatial ten feet wide. The house bore a startling resemblance to the houses my brother and sister and I owned, even though none of us had ever seen this place. When I'd bought my old farmhouse in North Carolina, for example, the first thing I'd done was to add a replica of this porch. Similarly, my brother's and sister's Louisiana homes, although newly designed by architects, bore an uncanny resemblance to the old George homestead.

As my mother and I strolled through the garden, where roses, day lilies, iris, vitex and phlox still bloomed, my mother remarked, "Your great-grandmother Emma loved flowers." Wanting to keep a part of this, my heritage, I knelt down and dug out one of the iris pips.

Because I also wanted to preserve something from the inside of the house, before it crumbled and was lost to time, we gingerly explored the interior, noting the twenty-inch-wide virgin pine boards, the hand-hewn beams and the handmade clay bricks, each marked with a G. Then, in the bedroom, I discovered Emma's 1890s wallpaper—a floral motif, naturally, with a repeating pattern of large bouquets of ivory and pink roses. It was peeling off the pine boards, but still lovely after all this time, just like my great-grandmother's garden. I knew this was the memento I wanted to take with me. With the tiny penknife on my key ring, I carved off two square-foot pieces, one for me and one for my younger sister, Cindy.

Before we headed for home, Mom and I stood on that familiar front porch for a moment of silent leave-taking. At that instant, I felt very connected to my ancestors, as though there were invisible wires running between us, anchoring each successive generation to the earlier ones. However, on the drive home, I began to wonder if I weren't making too much of this family ties thing. Perhaps a penchant for wide porches was just a coincidence.

The next day, eager to share the story of this trip with

Cindy, I dropped by her house. I found her in the kitchen, happily perusing the materials she had bought on a recent trip to England in order to redecorate her home. We sat at the table together, and I told her about our great-grandparents' farmhouse with its verandah, floor-to-ceiling windows and high ceilings that had somehow found their way into the design of the homes of the Georges' great-grandchildren. We laughed about my muddying my dress in order to dig out a flower pip, and then I produced the little square of wallpaper I'd brought for her as a keepsake.

She appeared stunned, sitting stone-still and dead-quiet. I thought I had, in my big-sister way, offended her with my story. Then she reached into the box of her renovation materials and pulled out the rolls of newly purchased wallpaper from England. The design was exactly the same—the ivory-pink sprays and bouquets of roses were Emma's.

Emma's bouquets had found their way into the present.

Pamela George

Between the Lines

Love is something that you can leave behind when you die. It's that powerful.

Jolik (Fire) Lame Deer Rosebud Lakota

After a moving memorial service for my beloved father, Walter Rist, our family gathered at our childhood home to be with Mother. Memories of Dad whirled in my mind. I could see his warm, brown eyes and contagious smile. I envisioned all six-foot-four of him in hat and coat, headed to teach his classes at the college. Quickly, a new scene flashed in my mind of Dad in a T-shirt, swinging a baseball bat, hitting long flies to us kids on the front lawn, years ago.

But special memories couldn't push away the dark shadows of separation from the man we loved.

Later in the evening, while looking for something in a closet, we found a paper sack marked, "Charlotte's Scrapbook." Curious, I opened it. There it was—my "Inspiration from Here and There" scrapbook I had kept as a teenager. I had forgotten all about it until this moment when I leafed through the pages of pasted pictures from magazines and church bulletins. They were punctuated with clippings of famous quotes, Bible verses and poetry. *This was me as a teenager,* I thought. *My heart's desires.*

Then I saw something I'd never seen before—my father's handwriting penciled on page after page! My throat tightened as I read the little notes Dad had slipped in to communicate with me. They were love messages and words of wisdom. I had no idea when he had written these, but this was the day to find them!

On the first page, Dad wrote, "Life is never a burden if love prevails." My chin quivered. I trembled. I could hardly believe the timeliness of his words. I flipped the pages for more.

Under a picture of a bride being given away by her father, my dad wrote, "How proud I was to walk down the aisle with you, Charlotte!"

Near a copy of the Lord's Prayer, he had scrawled, "I have always found the strength I needed, but only with God's help." What a comfort!

I turned to a picture of a young boy sitting on the grass with a gentle collie resting its head on his lap. Beneath it were these words: "I had a collie like this one when I was a boy. She was run over by a streetcar and disappeared. Three weeks later she came home, limping with a broken leg, her tail cut off. Her name was Queenie. She lived for many more years. I watched her give birth to seven puppies. I loved her very much. Dad."

My moist eyes blurred as I read another page. "Dear Charlotte, listen to your children! Let them talk. Never brush them aside. Never consider their words trivial. Hold Bob's hand whenever you can. Hold your children's hands. Much love will be transferred, much warmth to remember." What a treasure of guidance for me as a wife and mother! I clung to the words from my dad whose gentle big hand often had held mine.

In those moments of paging through the scrapbook, incredible comfort was etched on the gray canvas of my life. On this, the day my father was buried, he had a loving "last word." Such a precious surprise, somehow allowed by God, cast victorious light on the shadows of my grief. I was able to walk on, covered by fresh beacons of strength.

Charlotte Adelsperger

Bean Talk

Both the happiest and most contented moments of my childhood were spent in the company of my grand-mother, Dee-Dee. She was my confidante, friend and advisor. Whenever I think about her, I picture her in the kitchen, with me by her side, as she taught me the art of homemaking. My favorite activity was snapping green beans. We snapped beans to boil with onion, salt, pepper and a ham hock. This was her way; this was her mother's way. Bean-snapping was tedious but never boring. It pro-vided me with an opportunity to have her all to myself. She was a captive audience for my stories, thoughts, ideas, jokes and the ever-present analysis of my life.

In her kitchen, we each had our own stool at the bar that separated the kitchen from the dining room. Having my own distinct seat made me feel secure. Our conversa-tions over the beans were varied throughout the years: We talked about family, the death of my father, my first kiss, first date, engagement, marriage and children. We also talked about sunsets, her garden, the sound of rain, which comforted us both, and the feeling of grass, as we were both happier when we were barefoot. Sometimes we were simply silent, enjoying each other's companionship and nothing more; sometimes there was no need for words. And we laughed. We laughed until we cried. My childhood, adolescence and early adulthood were all scrutinized and enjoyed over beans.

During those moments of snapping, I felt nourished by the smells in the kitchen and the warmth of her touch when her hand would brush mine in the pursuit of beans. She listened to me. She loved me.

Suddenly, so it seemed, Dee-Dee was diagnosed with lung cancer and died within three months. I was faced with filling her unfillable shoes. I was lost. I was not ready for her to die because I was not grown yet. Although I was twenty-eight, I still needed her.

Two months after her death, I found myself snapping green beans. On my stool. In her house. Alone. My grandfather had requested the roast beef and green bean dinner. I knew he wanted her smell, her cooking, to feel her in the house. I did, too. He was in his usual spot, in his room watching sports on television. My husband and daughter Kristina were in the den, watching a movie, and I was alone. Suddenly, I was cold, too; I trembled, and I started to cry. I wept softly in front of my silent, stringy green witnesses. I did not yet realize why I was crying. How silly to cry in front of a bunch of beans!

Then, I noticed the silence, the devastating silence that an absent life leaves behind. This was the calm after the storm, after the frantic months of sickness, days of desperate burial procedures, and weeks of confusion and shock that followed. This was the moment that it all became real. The beans were only a catalyst for comprehension and clarity. Now what would I do? How could I, by myself, do what Dee-Dee and I had done together for over twenty years? I missed her. I had not grieved since the initial diagnosis. I had been so busy taking care of her and burying her that I did not have time to miss her. I had been a steamroller of strength, protecting her, guiding her and listening to her, just as she had been for me. And now I was utterly alone, and all because of the damn beans.

At that moment, Kristina bounced into the room with all of the enthusiasm that a six-year-old should have. At the sight of the beans, her eyes brightened and she said, "Oh Mommy, can I help you?"

Wallowing in my grief, I shook my head and said, "Honey, you don't know how to snap beans."

She replied, "But Mom, Dee-Dee taught me how!" I did not immediately remember Dee-Dee teaching her. Kristina saw my lack of understanding and pursued her case.

She explained, "Remember Mommy? Dee-Dee was sick on her couch when she taught me."

In an instant, my mind brought forth the memory. Just three months earlier, a couple of weeks before the cancer invaded her bones, Dee-Dee insisted that I bring a pan full of fresh green beans to her bedroom. She snapped those beans while lying on her couch, propped on one elbow. She was a skeleton; she had an oxygen tank, but she was teaching Kristina. At the time, I thought my grandmother was trying to be useful, attempting to maintain her control in an uncontrollable situation. I was wrong. She was leaving her legacy and giving Kristina her inheritance.

I said to Kristina, "Okay, honey. I forgot Dee-Dee taught you. Here, you can help me."

She smiled and said, "Thanks, Mommy." With that, she jumped into Dee-Dee's chair, grabbed a handful of beans, and began to tell me about her tree-climbing adventures.

I do not cry for Dee-Dee anymore. She is still with me. Her spirit surrounds me. Her whispered wisdom breezes through me and into Kristina. There is no end to life, only continuity. And a lot of beans to snap.

Veronica Hilton

A Legacy in a Soup Pot

Have you ever noticed the busier your life seems to be, the more empty it appears to become? I remember staring at my date book early one Monday morning—scores of meetings, deadlines and projects leered back at me, assailing my senses and demanding my attention. I remember thinking for the umpteenth time, *What does all this really matter?*

And lately, with all this introspection, I had been remembering my beloved grandmother. Gram had a sixth-grade education, an abundance of kitchen-table wisdom and a wonderful sense of humor. Everyone who met her thought it was so appropriate that she had been born on April 1—the day of practical jokes, good laughs and hearty humor—and she certainly spent her lifetime buoying up everyone's spirits.

Cerebral she was not, but to a child, she was Disney World personified. Every activity with Gram became an event, an occasion to celebrate, a reason to laugh. Looking back, I realize it was a different time, a different sphere. Family, fun and food played an important role.

Meals were Gram's mainstay—occasions to be planned,

savored and enjoyed. Hot, sit-down breakfasts were mandatory. The preparation of lunch began at 10:30 every morning, with homemade soup simmering, and dinner plans started at 3:30 P.M., with a telephone call to the local butcher to make a delivery. Gram spent a lifetime meeting the most basic needs of her family.

Stopping to pick up yet another take-out meal for dinner, my mind traveled back to her kitchen. The old, oak kitchen table, with the single pedestal . . . the endless pots of soups, stews and gravies perpetually simmering on the stove top . . . the homey tablecloths stained with love from a meal past. *My gosh*, I thought with a start. *I'm over forty, and I have yet to make a pot of soup or stew from scratch!*

Suddenly the cardboard take-out containers next to me looked almost obscene. I felt as if I had been blessed with a wonderful legacy, and for one reason or another, I had never quite gotten to the point of passing it on.

The following day, I rummaged through the attic searching for a cardboard box that had been stowed away. Twenty-five years ago, that box had been given to me when Gram decided to move from the old homestead. I vaguely remember going through my "inheritance" as a teen. Every granddaughter had received a pocketbook. Mine was a jeweled evening bag, circa 1920. I remembered I carried it at my college graduation. However, being a headstrong teen at the time of my "inheritance," I never really bothered with the rest of the contents. They remained sealed in that same box, buried somewhere in the attic.

It wasn't that difficult to locate the box, and it was even easier to open it. The tape was old and gave way easily. Lifting the top, I saw Gram had wrapped some items in old linen napkins—a butter dish, vase and at the bottom, one of her old soup pots. The lid was taped to the pot itself. I peeled back the tape and removed the lid.

At the bottom of the pot was a letter, penned in Gram's own hand:

My darling Barbara,

I know you will find this one day many years from now. While you are reading this, please remember how much I loved you, for I'll be with the angels then, and I won't be able to tell you myself.

You were always so headstrong, so quick, so much in a hurry to grow up. I often had wished that I could have kept you a baby forever. When you stop running, when it's time for you to slow down, I want you to take out your Gram's old soup pot and make your house a home. I have enclosed the recipe for your favorite soup, the one I used to make for you when you were my baby.

Remember I love you, and love is forever.

Your Gram

I sat reading that note over and over that morning, sobbing that I had not appreciated her enough when I had her. *You were such a treasure,* I moaned inwardly. *Why didn't I even bother to look inside this pot while you were still alive!*

So that night, my briefcase remained locked, the answering machine continued to blink and the disasters of the outside world were put on hold. I had a pot of soup to make.

Barbara Davey

More Chicken Soup?

Many of the stories and poems you have read in this book were submitted by readers like you who had read earlier *Chicken Soup for the Soul* books. We publish at least five or six *Chicken Soup for the Soul* books every year. We invite you to contribute a story to one of these future volumes.

Stories may be up to 1,200 words and must uplift or inspire. You may submit an original piece or something you clip out of the local newspaper, a magazine, a church bulletin or a company newsletter. It could also be your favorite quotation you've put on your refrigerator door or a personal experience that has touched you deeply.

To obtain a copy of our submission guidelines and a listing of upcoming *Chicken Soup* books, please write, fax or check one of our Web sites.

Chicken Soup for the Soul
P.O. Box 30880 • Santa Barbara, CA 93130, U.S.A.
fax: (001) 805-563-2945
To e-mail or visit our Web sites:
www.chickensoup.com
www.clubchickensoup.com

Just send a copy of your stories and other pieces to any of the above addresses.

We will be sure that both you and the author are credited for your submission.

For information about speaking engagements, other books, audiotapes, workshops and training programs, please contact any of the authors directly.

Supporting Women of the World

In the spirit of supporting women everywhere, the publisher and coauthors of *A Second Chicken Soup for the Woman's Soul* will donate a portion of the proceeds from this book to the YWCA of the U.S.A.

The YWCA is a nonprofit organization dedicated to the support and advancement of women and girls throughout the nation. Located in all fifty states, the YWCA is the largest provider of:

- Shelter services for women and children
- Quality, low-cost child care services
- Referral, screening and education services for breast and cervical cancer to low-income women over the age of fifty
- Public education campaigns to promote racial equality and understanding
- Youth services, including sports and fitness programs, mentoring programs to develop technological skills, and teen clubs to develop leadership

For more information, please contact this organization at:

YWCA of the U.S.A.
350 Fifth Avenue
New York, NY 10118, U.S.A.
tel: (001) 800-821-4364
or (001) 212-273-7800
Web Page: *www.ywca.org*

Who Is Jack Canfield?

Jack Canfield is one of America's leading experts in the development of human potential and personal effectiveness. He is both a dynamic, entertaining speaker and a highly sought-after trainer. Jack has a wonderful ability to inform and inspire audiences toward increased levels of self-esteem and peak performance.

He is the author and narrator of several bestselling audio- and videocassette programs, including *Self-Esteem and Peak Performance, How to Build High Self-Esteem, Self-Esteem in the Classroom* and *Chicken Soup for the Soul—Live.* He is regularly seen on television shows such as *Good Morning America, 20/20* and *NBC Nightly News.* Jack has coauthored numerous books, including the *Chicken Soup for the Soul* series, *Dare to Win* and *The Aladdin Factor* (all with Mark Victor Hansen), *100 Ways to Build Self-Concept in the Classroom* (with Harold C. Wells) and *Heart at Work* (with Jacqueline Miller).

Jack is a regularly featured speaker for professional associations, school districts, government agencies, churches, hospitals, sales organizations and corporations. His clients have included the American Dental Association, the American Management Association, AT&T, Campbell Soup, Clairol, Domino's Pizza, GE, ITT, Hartford Insurance, Johnson & Johnson, the Million Dollar Roundtable, NCR, New England Telephone, Re/Max, Scott Paper, TRW and Virgin Records. Jack is also on the faculty of Income Builders International, a school for entrepreneurs.

Jack conducts an annual eight-day Training of Trainers program in the areas of self-esteem and peak performance. It attracts educators, counselors, parenting trainers, corporate trainers, professional speakers, ministers and others interested in developing their speaking and seminar-leading skills.

For further information about Jack's books, tapes and training programs, or to schedule him for a presentation, please contact:

The Canfield Training Group
P.O. Box 30880 • Santa Barbara, CA 93130, U.S.A.
phone: (001) 805-563-2935 • fax: (001) 805-563-2945
To e-mail or visit our Web site:
www.chickensoup.com

Who Is Mark Victor Hansen?

Mark Victor Hansen is a professional speaker who, in the last twenty years, has made over four-thousand presentations to more than 2 million people in thirty-two countries. His presentations cover sales excellence and strategies; personal empowerment and development; and how to triple your income and double your time off.

Mark has spent a lifetime dedicated to his mission of making a profound and positive difference in people's lives. Throughout his career, he has inspired hundreds of thousands of people to create a more powerful and purposeful future for themselves while stimulating the sale of billions of dollars worth of goods and services.

Mark is a prolific writer and has authored *Future Diary, How to Achieve Total Prosperity* and *The Miracle of Tithing.* He is coauthor of the *Chicken Soup for the Soul* series, *Dare to Win* and *The Aladdin Factor* (all with Jack Canfield) and *The Master Motivator* (with Joe Batten).

Mark has also produced a complete library of personal empowerment audio- and videocassette programs that have enabled his listeners to recognize and use their innate abilities in their business and personal lives. His message has made him a popular television and radio personality, with appearances on ABC, NBC, CBS, HBO, PBS and CNN. He has also appeared on the cover of numerous magazines, including *Success, Entrepreneur* and *Changes.*

Mark is a big man with a heart and spirit to match—an inspiration to all who seek to better themselves.

For further information about Mark write:

P.O. Box 7665
Newport Beach, CA 92658, U.S.A.
phone: (001) 949-759-9304 or (001) 800-433-2314
fax: (001) 949-722-6912
Web site: *www.chickensoup.com*

Who Is Jennifer Read Hawthorne?

Jennifer Read Hawthorne is coauthor of the #1 *New York Times* best-sellers *Chicken Soup for the Woman's Soul* and *Chicken Soup for the Mother's Soul*. Currently at work on future *Chicken Soup for the Soul* books, she also delivers *Chicken Soup for the Soul* presentations nationwide, sharing inspirational stories of love and hope, courage and dreams.

Jennifer is known as a dynamic and insightful speaker, with a great sense of humor and a gift for telling stories. From an early age she developed a deep appreciation for language, cultivated by her parents. She attributes her love of storytelling to the legacy of her late father, Brooks Read, a renowned Master Storyteller whose original Brer Rabbit stories filled her childhood with magic and a sense of the power of words.

As a Peace Corps volunteer in West Africa teaching English as a foreign language, Jennifer discovered the universality of stories to teach, move, uplift and connect people. Her *Chicken Soup for the Soul* presentations make audiences laugh and cry; many people say their lives are changed for the better as a result of hearing her speak.

Jennifer is cofounder of The Esteem Group, a company specializing in self-esteem and inspirational programs for women. A professional speaker since 1975, she has spoken to thousands of people around the world about personal growth, self-development and professional success. Her clients have included professional associations, Fortune 500 companies, and government and educational organizations such as AT&T, Delta Airlines, Hallmark Cards, The American Legion, Norand, Cargill, the State of Iowa and Clemson University.

Jennifer is a native of Baton Rouge, Louisiana, where she graduated from Louisiana State University with a degree in journalism. She lives in Fairfield, Iowa, with her husband, Dan, and two stepchildren, Amy and William.

If you would like to schedule Jennifer for a *Chicken Soup for the Soul* keynote address or seminar, you may contact her at:

Jennifer Hawthorne Inc.
1105 South D Street
Fairfield, IA 52556, U.S.A.
phone: (001) 515-472-7136 • fax: (001) 515-469-6908

Who Is Marci Shimoff?

Marci Shimoff is coauthor of the #1 *New York Times* bestsellers *Chicken Soup for the Woman's Soul* and *Chicken Soup for the Mother's Soul.* She is also a professional speaker and trainer who, for the last seventeen years, has inspired thousands of people with her message of personal and professional growth. She gives seminars and keynote addresses on self-esteem, stress management, communication skills and peak performance. Since 1994, she has specialized in delivering *Chicken Soup for the Soul* keynote addresses to audiences around the world.

Marci is cofounder and president of The Esteem Group, a company that offers self-esteem and inspirational programs for women. As a top-rated speaker for Fortune 500 companies, Marci's clients have included AT&T, General Motors, Sears, Amoco, American Airlines and Bristol-Myers Squibb. She has also been a featured speaker for numerous professional organizations, universities and women's associations, where she is known for her lively humor and her dynamic delivery.

Marci combines her energetic style with a strong knowledge base. She earned her MBA from UCLA; she also studied for one year in the U.S. and Europe to earn an advanced certificate as a stress-management consultant. Since 1989, Marci has studied self-esteem with Jack Canfield, and has assisted in his annual Training of Trainers program for professionals.

In 1983, Marci coauthored a highly acclaimed study of the fifty top business women in America. Since that time, she has specialized in addressing women's audiences, focusing on helping women discover the extraordinary within themselves.

Of all the projects Marci has worked on in her career, none have been as fulfilling as creating *Chicken Soup for the Soul* books. Currently at work on future editions of *Chicken Soup for the Soul,* she is thrilled at the opportunity to help touch the hearts and rekindle the spirits of millions of people throughout the world.

If you would like to schedule Marci for a *Chicken Soup for the Soul* keynote address or seminar, you can reach her at:

The Esteem Group
191 Bayview Drive
San Rafael, CA 94901, U.S.A.
phone: (001) 415-789-1300 • fax: (001) 415-789-1309

Contributors

Susan Adair is a social worker for the Texas Department of Human Services. She lives in Lufkin, Texas, with her husband, John and their two daughters.

Denaé Adams lives in Bethel, Ohio. She is a graduate of Morehead State University in Kentucky and did her student teaching in England, working with students with severe emotional, behavioral and learning disorders. During her stay, she had the opportunity to travel to France, Belgium, Scotland and Holland. She is now a teacher for students with severe emotional and behavioral disorders in Ripley, Ohio.

Charlotte Adelsperger is an inspirational freelance writer and speaker. She is the author of two books, and has written for over seventy publications. She enjoys speaking on ways to encourage others. She is thankful for her husband, Bob and grown children, Karen Hayse and John Adelsperger—creative "cheerleaders" in her life. Charlotte can be reached at 11629 Riley, Overland Park, KS 66210, or by calling 913-345-1678.

Carol Allen is a professional Vedic astrologer living in the beautiful wilderness of northern New Mexico with her husband, Bill, and her tabby cat, Buddha. She also has a story in *Hot Chocolate for the Mystical Soul* and is writing a comedic book about animals. You can reach her by calling 505-737-2398.

Shirley Allison is an avid antique collector who runs an antique shop with her husband Dan. She is the mother of two and the grandmother of six who most values the close knit relationship she enjoys with her family. She urges people to contact the National Kidney Foundation at 1-800-622-9010 to find out more about the life-saving benefits of organ donation. Shirley asks, "Please don't put it off, do it today!"

Helen Troisi Arney and her husband Paul, transplanted Pennsylvanians, spent their married life of forty-three-plus years in Peoria, Illinois, rearing three sons and three daughters. Helen earned B.A. and M.A. degrees at Bradley University and taught high school English for nineteen years. She has been published in newspapers and magazines, including *Chicago Tribune* magazine and *Reader's Digest*, and writes a column, "Widowed Walk" for the Peoria *Times Observer*. She can be reached at 8660 N. Picture Ridge Rd., Peoria, IL 61615.

Marsha Arons is a writer and lecturer in Skokie, Illinois. She is thrilled to be associated with the *Chicken Soup* series, and her stories appear in *Woman's Soul* and *Mother's Soul*. She also contributes to national magazines such as *Good Housekeeping*, *Reader's Digest* and *Redbook*. She has authored a book for young adults and is currently at work on a collection of short stories dealing with mother-daughter relationships. You can contact her via e-mail for speaking or other assignments at *RA8737@aol.com*.

Shinan Barclay is an award-winning author, poet and storyteller. She publishes *Humbug Mountain News, a Fairy Godmother's Journal of Miracles*,

Magic and Spiritual Midwifery. She is the coauthor of *The Sedona Vortex Experience* and *Flowering Woman Moontime for Kory*, the story of a girl's rite of passage into womanhood. She works as a midwife in Palliative Care "singing people over." You may contact her at *shinan_barclay@yahoo.com or at http://edgecity.com/shinanagans*.

Shirley Barksdale has been freelance writing since she lost her son in 1972. She wrote for Frontier Airlines for fourteen years and has written for several other publications including *Virtue* magazine, *Guideposts*, *Reader's Digest* and *McCall's*. She resides in Colorado with her husband, Ralph, who is a retired commercial airline pilot for United Airlines. Shirley may be reached at 11 Canongate Lane, Highlands Ranch, CO 80126.

Beverly Beckham is an award-winning columnist and editorial writer for *The Boston Herald*. She is the author of *A Gift of Time*, a collection of personal essays. An at-home mother who embarked upon a writing career at age thirty, she routinely ponders the universal experiences that connect family and friends. You can reach her at P.O. Box 216, Canton, MA 02021, or by e-mailing her at *BevBeckham@aol.com*.

Randy Bisson is a professional cartoonist who has been selling cartoons to magazines and books since 1973. He has sold to hundreds of different magazines including *Better Homes & Gardens*, *Good Housekeeping*, *Saturday Evening Post*, *Woman's World* and *First for Women*.

Sally A. Breslin is a newspaper correspondent and photographer for Neighborhood Publications Inc. in Bedford, New Hampshire. Since 1994, she also has been writing a weekly humor column, "My Life," for which she was named the 1995 Columnist of the Year by the New Hampshire Press Association. Her column also can be seen weekly on *www.NH.com*. She has had articles published in *The Writer*, *Datebook* and *NH Home* magazines. In her free time, Breslin enjoys analyzing people's dreams, which she does on-air monthly at WJYY Radio in Concord, New Hampshire. You can reach her at P.O. Box 585, Suncook, NH 03275-0585.

Gina Bridgeman is a regular contributor to the devotional book *Daily Guideposts* and writes for *Guideposts* magazine. She is also a consulting editor to the Fellowship of Merry Christians' *Joyful Noiseletter*. Gina lives in Scottsdale, Arizona, with her husband and two children.

Jean Brody is a national magazine columnist, Kentucky newspaper columnist, and public motivational speaker. She has published over thirty short stories, articles and poems nationally and is the author of the book, *Braille Me: A Beyond Seeing Experience*. She lives on a Kentucky farm with her husband Gene, one dog, two cats, one goat and horses. She can be reached at 606-745-4779.

Marty Bucella has had over 10,000 cartoons published in more than 400 magazines both here and abroad. His work can regularly be seen in *Better Homes & Gardens*, *Woman's World*, *The National Enquirer*, etc. The artist's work can be seen on greeting cards, T-shirts, calendars, textbooks and in newspapers through syndication. Marty can be reached at *MJBTOONS@aol.com.*

Isabel Bearman Bucher, a recently retired fifth grade teacher and first generation Italian American, was born in Branford, Connecticut in 1937. Raised in small town U.S.A., she was peppered with the richness of her family including strong female figures. At twenty-seven, in 1965, she married LeRoy Bearman, an Albuquerque sports journalist and had two daughters, Erica and Shauna, melding her background to LeRoy's Jewish one. His untimely death at forty-two, of cardiovascular disease set her on a new course of rebuilding. Happily remarried now for almost twenty years to Robert, a retired banker, she and her now-grown daughters continue the tradition of The Melding.

Cindy Jevne Buck is a professional writer and writing instructor who is currently collecting heartwarming stories for a book about gardening. She is still good friends with the star of her story, Michael MacCallum, who lives in Ashby, Massachusetts. You can reach Cindy at 51 N. Cromwell St., Fairfield, IA 52556, or by fax or phone at 515-472-6022.

Martha Campbell is a graduate of Washington University School of Fine Arts, and a former writer-designer for Hallmark Cards. Since she became a freelancer in 1973, she has had over 20,000 cartoons published and has illustrated nineteen books. You can write her at P.O. Box 2538, Harrison, AR 72602 or call 870-741-5323.

Dave Carpenter has been a full-time cartoonist and humorous illustrator since 1981. His cartoons have appeared in *Barrons, The Wall Street Journal, Forbes, Better Homes & Gardens, Good Housekeeping, Woman's World, First, The Saturday Evening Post* and numerous other publications. Dave can be reached at P.O. Box 520, Emmetsburg, IA 50536, or by calling 712-852-3725.

Sharon M. Chamberlain is an artist, writer, mother and grandmother. "Color My World" is a snippet from her autobiography which she began writing after becoming disabled. Sharon also enjoys incorporating her poetry and prose into her original watercolors. She can be contacted at 4315 N. University, Peoria, IL 61614, or by calling 309-686-1568.

Dan Clark is the international ambassador of the "Art of Being Alive." He has spoken to over 2 million people in all fifty states, Canada, Europe, Asia and Russia. Dan is an actor, songwriter, recording artist, video producer and award-winning athlete. He is the well-known author of six books, including *Getting High—How to Really Do It, One Minute Messages, Puppies for Sale,* and *The Art of Being Alive.* He can be reached at P.O. Box 8689, Salt Lake City, UT 84108 or call 801-485-5755.

Teresa Collins lives in Chelsea, Oklahoma, with her husband and three sons. She is the author of her low-fat cookbook, *Low Fat & Happy.* In it, you will find over two hundred easy-to-follow recipes along with her secrets to getting motivated. Remember, you are worth not giving up on. You can reach her at

Aspire Publications, P.O. Box 392, Chelsea, OK 74016, or by calling 918-789-2765.

Robert A. Concolino has specialized in family law for twenty-five years. He advocates alternatives to adversarial win-lose tactics of judging and blaming to create freedom and power of responsible choices. For information about his workshops and consultations, write to 17602 17th Street, #102-113, Tustin, CA 92780, or call 888-TRUEWIN.

George Crenshaw is an old pro with a long track record of success. He is an ex-Walt Disney animator, a magazine cartoonist with top sales to top slicks for three decades, the creator of *NUBBIN* by King Features, creator of *GUMDROP* by United Features, creator of the *MUFFINS* by Columbia Features, creator of *BELVEDERE* by Post Dispatch Features and the President of Post Dispatch Features, Masters Agency, Inc.

Barbara Davey is the director of marketing and public relations at Christ Hospital in Jersey City, New Jersey. She received bachelor's and master's degrees from Seton Hall University. A project dear to her heart is "The Look Good, Feel Better" program, which helps women undergoing chemotherapy and radiation for cancer cope with the unpleasant cosmetic side effects of their treatments by providing wigs and make-overs. She and her husband, Reinhold Becker, live in Verona, New Jersey. You can reach her by calling 973-239-6568.

Mary J. Davis began writing when the "empty nest" syndrome hit home. Mary specializes in Christian education, writing, inspirational writing and children's fiction with over 200 articles in print. Her twenty books have been published by Rainbow Legacy and Shining Star. She speaks at Christian Education seminars, ladies' groups and children's rallies. She also presents writing workshops for children. Mary and husband, Larry, have three grown children. You can reach her at P.O. Box 27, Montrose, IA 52639.

Drue Duke is a freelance writer, experienced in radio, stage and magazine writing. Her emphasis is on Christian and inspirational subjects. Her book, *Alabama Tales: Anecdotes, Legends and Other Stories,* can be ordered from Vision Press, P.O. Box 1106, Northport, AL 35476. She may be contacted at 256-381-0829.

Ron C. Eggertsen grew up in Southern California and was educated at Brigham Young University and the University of Southern California. He has been a Naval officer, advertising executive, television writer, radio announcer, communications consultant, documentary film producer and is working on becoming a "whole human being." He lives in Orem, Utah, and can be reached at 801-224-2257, or *rone@burgoyne.com.*

Lin Faubel has three sons, one daughter, two grandsons and three ex-husbands. To balance her chaotic personal life, she has started a business organizing homes for sale. Her mind and body reside in Illinois, while her heart and soul live in a lighthouse in New England. Lin may be reached at 111 S. Lawndale, Washington, IL 61571, or call 309-444-8253.

Arnold Fine has been the senior editor of THE JEWISH PRESS, the largest

Anglo Jewish Newspaper in the world, for forty-eight years. At the same time he was coordinator of special education at Samuel J. Tilden High School in Brooklyn, caring for handicapped and brain injured children. Since retiring from the school system Mr. Fine has become an adjunct professor in the behavioral science department at Kingsborough College. He has been honored by the National Committee for the Furtherance of Jewish Education and the Jewish Teachers Association of New York State. He was nominated twice as the "Teacher of The Year" in New York State. He is married, has three sons and six grandchildren.

Lisa Marie Finley is a first-grade teacher and wife and mother of two young sons. She keeps very busy. But frequently a poem or short story will come to mind, is finished in moments, and is gone just as quickly if not written down. In these moments, there is yet another, special kind of "full"fillment. You can reach her at P.O. Box 536, Stanwood, WA 98292.

Barbara Jeanne Fisher resides in Fremont, Ohio. Ms. Fisher is a prolific writer and has published numerous articles in magazines throughout the United States and Canada. Although fictional, in her first novel, *Stolen Moments*, to be released in October, 1998, many of the emotions portrayed by the characters come from her experience in dealing with lupus in her own life. Her goal in writing the book was to use the feelings of her heart to touch the hearts of others.

George M. Flynn is a freelance writer and seventh-grade English teacher at Frankford Township School in Branchville, New Jersey. He resides with his wife, Carole, and their three children, Jeannie, Katie and Jimmy at 23 Kemah-Mecca Lake Road, Newton, NJ 07860. You can reach him by calling 973-948-4995. "Veronica's Babies" first appeared in the fall 1997 issue of *Vermont Ink*.

Toni Fulco has authored over 150 articles, stories and poems in national magazines and anthologies. She raises cockatiels at home and is known locally as "the bird lady" for her affectionate, talkative, hand-fed baby birds. You can reach her at 89 Penn Estates, E. Stroudsburg, PA 18301.

Deb Plouse Fulton is in her twenty-second year of teaching elementary-aged learning disabled children. She resides with husband, Steve, and her three children: Jori (seventeen), Jena (sixteen) and Jacob (nine). You can reach her at 16 Hillcrest Drive, Middletown, PA 17057.

Mechi Garza, a Choctaw-Cherokee Elder, is active with various intertribal groups, serves on the Elder's Council and is the Spiritual Counselor for Native Americans at a Federal Prison. Her twenty grandchildren represent five different races. She has written eleven books and is a member of the International Women's Writers Guild. A television documentary of her life is to be released soon.

Pamela George is a professor of educational psychology at North Carolina Central University. She researches and writes about how children think and learn across cultures. She lives with her husband and daughter in Durham, North Carolina.

Frankie Germany has a master's degree in elementary education and has taught for twenty-seven years. Her writing has come about late in life but she plans to continue for as long as she lives. She looks forward to the time when she can write full time. Frankie and her husband have a blended family of six children and two beautiful grandchildren.

Evelyn M. Gibb, after raising three children, now lives with her husband in the foothills of Washington's Cascade Mountains. Her great joys come from the natural beauty around her and sharing her short stories, articles and poems with readers of many national magazines. She recently completed a book-length, true chronicle of an early bicycle adventure in 1909, *Two Bikes and a Billiken*.

Jean Jeffrey Gietzen is a poet and essayist whose family pieces have appeared in *McCall's, Reader's Digest, Writer's Digest* and *Catholic Digest* and many small press magazines. Of her writings, Jean says, "Writing about family, its ups and its downs, is a way to help others see they are not alone in resolving issues that arise in any loving family. It's a way to touch hearts and perhaps do some healing along the way." Jean is a former Midwesterner who now writes from her retirement nest in Tucson, Arizona where she occasionally teaches writing classes. Mother of three, grandmother of four, she is also the author of *A People Set Apart* and *Questions and Answers for Catechists*. Her work has also been featured in Multnomah's *Stories from the Heart* line. Jean can be reached at 520-296-1550.

Randy Glasbergen is the creator of the cartoon *The Better Half* which is syndicated to 150 newspapers by King Features Syndicate. More than 20,000 of Randy's cartoons have been published in magazines, books and greeting cards around the world. Look for Randy's daily cartoons online at *www.norwich.net/~randyg/toon.html*.

Barbara E. C. Goodrich, originally from Valparaiso, Indiana, is a freelance writer currently living in the beautiful rainforests of Australia. Her experience in the personal development industry has given her unique insights in teaching life-story writing workshops. She can be reached at: P.O. Box 84, Tyalgum, NSW, 2484, Australia.

Patrick Hardin is a cartoonist and illustrator whose work has appeared in a variety of books and periodicals around the world. He currently enjoys the urban grit of his home town Flint, Michigan. You may reach him at 134 Commonwealth Ave., Flint, MI 48503, by calling 810-234-7452 or faxing 810-233-7531.

Jonny Hawkins is a nationally known cartoonist whose work has appeared in *The Saturday Evening Post, National Enquirer, Barron's* and over 175 other publications. His syndicated comic feature *Hi and Jinx* runs in many U.S. newspapers.

Donna Kay Heath is the mother of one daughter and is a Christian writer and speaker. She recently published a book of poetry and has spoken to various women's groups. "My desire is to encourage those who are hurting from life's struggles. I'm proof we can get through them and become stronger because of them." For speaking or purchase of her book, *From the Heart,* she can be reached at 910-259-2243 or at Bridge Builders Ministry, P.O. Box 1146, Burgaw, NC 28425.

Jacqueline M. Hickey is a freelance writer living in Rockport, Massachusetts, with her husband and three children. Currently working on her first novel, Jacqueline is continually inspired by the pristine beauty of Rockport. She can be reached at 6½ R. Parker Street, Rockport, MA 01966, or by e-mail at *bojack@tiac.net.*

Caroline Castle Hicks is a former high school English and humanities teacher who is now a stay-at-home mother, freelance writer and poet. She lives in Huntersville, North Carolina, where she derives great inspiration from her family and from the abundant natural beauty of her native state. Her e-mail address is *Dhicks1@compuserve.com.*

Veronica Hilton is a mother (of eight-year-old Kristina), writer, wife and student. After traveling the states and Europe with her now-retired Air Force husband, Richard, the thirty-year-old, Southern-influenced poet (Tennessee born and a Florida transplant) returned to academics, currently attending Florida Atlantic University. Veronica devotes her time to Girl Scout leadership and academic honor societies. You can reach her at 940 39th Court, West Palm Beach, FL 33407, or by calling 561-465-0838.

Geery Howe, president of Morning Star Associates, is a consultant, speaker and trainer in leadership, management and strategic development. He is the author of *Listen to the Heart: The Transformational Pathway to Health and Wellness* and can be reached at Morning Star Associates, P.O. Box 869, West Branch, IA 52358, or by calling 319-643-2257.

Steven James is a dynamic speaker, writer and educator who travels the country inspiring listeners with his animated messages and engaging true stories. His articles regularly appear in leading Christian magazines and share the relevance of God's love for people of today. To book Steven for your next retreat, conference or seminar, write to him at P.O. Box 141, Johnson City, TN 37605, e-mail him at *storyguy@pobox.com,* or call him at 800-527-8679.

Kitsy Jones is first and foremost a wife and mother who loves spending time with her family. Her children are now seven and eleven and she and Lee have been married for fifteen years. She is a registered nurse who works at Cook Children's Medical Center in Fort Worth, specializing in bone marrow transplantation. She feels blessed to have witnessed this special Christmas miracle. She can be reached at P.O. Box 15201, Arlington, TX 76015 or e-mail at *Isjones1@airmail. net.*

Bil Keane draws the internationally syndicated cartoon *The Family Circus* which appears in more than 1,500 newspapers. Created in 1960, it is based on

Keane's own family: his wife, Thel and their five children. Now nine grand-children provide most of the inspirations.

Harrison Kelly lives in Memphis, Tennessee with his wife of sixteen years and their two children, Brad and Kristina. Currently, he is seeking agent representation for his first novel and is working on a suspense thriller. He can be reached via e-mail at *dhk@sprynet.com*. "Not-So-White . . ." is his first published story.

Sue Monk Kidd is the bestselling author of six books of spirituality, including *When the Heart Waits* and her highly acclaimed spiritual memoir *The Dance of the Dissident Daughter* (Harper San Francisco). A lecturer and teacher, she has published hundreds of essays and articles in publications such as *Reader's Digest, Weavings, Guideposts* and *The Atlanta Journal Constitution*. Her fiction has been published in literary journals and received numerous awards, including a Katherine Anne Porter Award and citations from Best American Short Stories.

Marilyn King is a two-time Olympian (1972/1976) in the grueling five-event pentathlon. An automobile accident rendered her unable to train physically for her third Olympic Team. Using only mental rehearsal, she placed second at the trials for the Moscow Games. Marilyn is now an internationally acclaimed business consultant, inspirational speaker and trainer who assists participants in discovering how profoundly their thinking affects their health, their performance and their future. You may contact her at 484-149 Lake Park Ave., Oakland, CA 94610, or by calling 510-568-7417, or by e-mailing her at *Olympianmk@aol.com*.

Lynne Kinghorn resides with her husband in Denver, where she is a licensed clinical psychologist in private practice. A nationally-published freelancer, she writes extensively on mothers' self-esteem issues. She also developed and presents the business seminar, "How to Tame an Angry Customer," and is working on her first novel. You can reach her at 1777 S. Bellaire Street, Suite 300, Denver, CO 80222, or by calling 303-757-5907.

Norma R. Larson was associate editor of a greeting card company who put her career on hold to actively participate in the pastoral ministry of her husband, Arthur, in churches in Connecticut and Illinois. After their three children left the nest to become a doctor, an educator and an attorney, she resumed writing and has published *Hospital Patience* (Revell), a balm for inner healing through generous doses of hope and humor. Recently widowed, she resides in Morton, Illinois.

Steven J. Lesko Jr. is a retired professor of civil technology from Monroe Community College in Rochester, New York, where he taught for thirty years and practiced civil engineering for sixteen years. He was married to a wonderful lady, who gave him great happiness, for over fifty years. They were blessed with three children, nine grandchildren and three great-grandchildren. Their strong Catholic faith has always been the center of their lives. You can reach him at 86 Highledge Drive, Penfield, NY 14526, or by calling 716-248-0496.

Helen Luecke is an inspirational writer of short stories, articles and devotionals. She helped organize Inspirational Writers Alive! (Amarillo chapter). You can reach her at 2921 S. Dallas, Amarillo, TX 79103, or by calling 806-376-9671.

Louisa Godissart McQuillen writes from her home in Chester Hill, a small town in Pennsylvania at the demarcation line between Clearfield and Centre County. Louisa has been writing since childhood and is published nationally and internationally. Contact her for future chapbooks at 525 Decatur St., Philipsburg, PA 16866, or e-mail her at *LZM4@PSU.EDU.*

Margaret McSherry was born in County Durham England. Her mother died when she was one year old. She was raised in Ireland from age three to fifteen. At fifteen her father sent her a ticket to join him in America. She married an American on December 7, 1941, Pearl Harbor Day. She worked for her living from her arrival in this country until she was forced to retire, by medical disabilities, at age sixty-one. She was seventy-seven years of age when the events in this story took place. Her two daughters, two sons-in law, six grandchildren and five great grandchildren are all very proud of her.

Joyce Meier's poems and short stories have been published in numerous literary magazines, including *Descant, Amelia* and *Riversedge.* One of her stories is included in the collection called *Common Bonds,* published by the SMU Press. For seven years she edited *Sands,* a literary magazine. She is currently working on her second novel.

Cynthia Mercati is a playwright and has twenty-two scripts published. She says, "As a professional actress, I currently perform with a children's theater company, often appearing in my own shows. As an essayist, I often write about my family and baseball. And as a Chicago White Sox fan, I've learned to live on faith, and hang my hat on hope." She can be reached at P.O. Box 208, Waukee, IA, 50263, or by calling 515-987-2587.

Roberta Messner, R.N., Ph.D., is the author of several books and approximately 1,000 articles and short stories which have appeared in over 100 different publications. She writes and speaks on a wide variety of inspirational, health care and home decorating topics. She can be reached at 6283 Aracoma Rd., Huntington, WV 25705, or by calling 304-733-5466.

Wendy Miles is a third generation Floridian. Her great grandfather came to Florida from Chicago in 1880 and she grew up on the Gulf Coast of Florida when the land was still covered with orange groves and pine woods. Wendy has lived in Europe, worked for the B.B.C., taught transcendental meditation, earned a Ph.D. in English literature and has been a college professor. Wendy and her daughter and their cat, Oreo, love movies and music. She is now a full-time writer and editor. You can reach her at *msmiles@kdsi.net* or at 515-472-7050.

Jacquelyn Mitchard is the author of the nationally acclaimed #1 bestselling novel *THE DEEP END OF THE OCEAN* (Viking), which has been sold in twenty-two countries around the world. It is soon to be released as a major motion picture, starring Michelle Pfeiffer. Mitchard is also, most recently, the author of a new novel, THE MOST WANTED (Viking), and THE REST OF US (Viking), a collection of her nationally syndicated newspaper columns. She lives in Madison, Wisconsin, with her husband and five children.

Jill Williford Mitchell grew up in Arlington, Texas. She holds degrees in English and law, and studied at the University of Paris, Sorbonne. Her publications include legal articles, a short story and two poems. She can be reached at 3811 LakeRidge Rd., Arlington, TX 76016, by calling 505-763-7720, or by e-mail at *jmmitchell@etsc.net.*

Sarah Ann Reeves Moody was born in Waynesville, North Carolina. Daughter of William and Nora Jean Reeves, she is the youngest of four children. She is married to David Ray Moody and has four children and four grandchildren. She resides in Hampton, Virginia.

Carla Muir is a freelance writer. Her stories and poetry have been published in *More Stories for the Heart, Do Not Lose Heart, A Joy I'd Never Known, Glimpses of Heaven, The Worth of a Man* and other publications. Carla may be contacted through Yates & Yates, L.L.P., at 714-285-9540.

Chris Mullins is president and founder of ABOVE & BEYOND, a communications and consulting firm which delivers no nonsense, high energy, interactive seminars, workshops and keynotes that deal with topics such as leadership, team building, customer service, sales, telemarketing and personal/professional growth. Mullins' has over fifteen years of experience in both reorganizing and creating successful sales and customer service departments. Call 603-924-1640, visit his Web site at *http://www.top.monad.net/users/aboveandbeyond,* e-mail him at *aboveandbeyond@monad.net,* or write to 6 Cheney Ave., Suite A, Peterborough, NH 03458.

Gerry Niskern is a Phoenix-based freelance writer whose stories evoke nostalgic memories. Her articles appear in the Phoenix Newspapers. Gerry is currently working on a memoir entitled, *Don't Throw the Bread!* She enjoys success as a professional artist. Her prints are distributed worldwide. Originals may be seen on *http://www.thegalleries.com.* She can be reached at 602-943-3530, faxed at 602-870-0770, or e-mailed at *niskern@juno.com.*

Diane Novinski is a widow who is dedicated to raising two happy, healthy children after experiencing the terror, sadness and pain of losing a husband to cancer. "Never, Never Give Up" is a true story written as a tribute to her husband, Ben. She lives in Old Saybrook, Connecticut.

Jerry Perkins is farm editor of *The Des Moines Register,* a position he has held since June, 1993. He was a reporter at the *Register* from 1978 to 1988 and was an agribusiness writer from 1982 to 1988. He was public affairs director of the Iowa Corn Growers Association-Iowa Corn Promotion Board from 1988 to 1993, and managed the Russian-American Agribusiness Center in Stavropal, Russia from May to December, 1992 while on a leave of absence from the Corn

Growers. He is a native of Des Moines, Iowa, graduated from George Washington University in 1970 and spent two years in the Peace Corps from 1970 to 1972, serving in Panama and Nicaragua. He and his wife, Peggy, have three sons and live in Des Moines.

Teresa Pitman is a writer specializing in parenting and children's issues. She is a coauthor of several books, including *Best Evidence,* a book about pregnancy and childbirth and *Steps and Stages,* a series of four books that are collections of magazine articles about children at different ages. All are published by HarperCollins. Teresa can be reached at 905-847-3206, 2526 Woburn Cresc., Oakville, Ontario, Canada L6L 5E9.

Elaine Pondant is a partner of Pondant Projects, a freelance writing business established with her sister over twelve years ago. Often tapping into their own experiences, their projects include novels, novelettes, educational books, how-to booklets and articles for the print media. You may reach Elaine at 3717 Standrige, Carrollton, TX 75007, or by calling 972-492-7637.

Carol A. Price-Lopata has been a speaker for fifteen years throughout the United States, Europe and Australia. She specializes in self-esteem building and *Becoming the Hero You Have Always Been.* She sells thousands of her tape, *21 Days to Self-Discovery,* and is available to speak to organizations and associations. She can be reached at P.O. Box 8731, Madeira Beach, FL 33738, by calling 813-397-9111, or by faxing 813-397-3661.

Carol McAdoo Rehme is an energetic mother of four and a freelance writer. She also channels her pursuits—reading, researching, writing and speaking—into a business passion: the tell-tale art of storytelling. She can be reached at 2503 Logan Drive, Loveland, CO 80538, or by calling 970-669-5791.

Betty Reid resides in Ellicott City, Maryland with her husband and son. Besides writing poetry, she enjoys reading, collecting antiques and traveling with family. Her family and friends are often the inspiration behind her poetry. Betty would welcome your call at 410-461-6951.

Dan Rosandich draws for publications nationwide including magazines, book publishers and newsletters, and will tackle any assignments. His work has appeared in *Saturday Evening Post* and *National Review.* Rosandich can be reached anytime, voice or fax, at 906-482-6234.

Gail Rosenblum is a writer, editor and mother of three who specializes in the fields of health and families. You can find more of Rosenblum's writing at *www.dealingwith.com,* a Web site that helps people find support when dealing with family, health and emotional issues, including grief, divorce, cancer, aging and dozens of other topics. E-mail her at: *grosenblum@dealingwith.com.*

Daniel Schantz is an education professor at Central Christian College in Moberly, Missouri. He is the author of *You Can Teach with Success* from Standard Publishing Co., and he is a frequent contributor to *Guideposts Magazine* and *The Lookout.* He and his wife, Sharon, are the parents of two journalist daughters,

Teresa Williams and Natalie Cleeton.

Shelley Peterman Schwarz, an award-winning writer and professional motivational speaker, has had multiple sclerosis since 1979. Her books include, *Blooming Where You're Planted: Stories from the Heart,* and three *Making Life Easier* books: *250 Tips for Arthritis, Dressing Tips and Clothing Resources,* and *The Best 25 Catalog Resources.* You can reach Shelley at 933 Chapel Hill Road, Madison, WI 53711, e-mail her at *help@MakingLifeEasier.com,* or visit her Web site at *http://www.MakingLifeEasier.com.*

Vahan Shirvanian went from Air Force gunnery instructor (World War II) to *Saturday Evening Post* cartoonist in 1946. He quickly became one of the world's bestselling cartoonists and three times has been voted Best Cartoonist of the Year. He can be reached at 44 Hanover Rd., Mountain Lakes, NJ 07046, or by calling 973-334-8998.

Deborah Shouse's parents always told her to "do the write thing." She has been trying ever since. Deborah is a writer, creativity consultant and speaker. Her writing has appeared in *Reader's Digest, Newsweek, Redbook* and *Ms.* She coauthored *Working Woman's Communications Survival Guide* (Prentice Hall). Deborah can be reached at The Write Stuff, 6619 Hodges, Prairie Village, KS 66208, by calling 913-671-7195, or by e-mailing her at *doidare@bigfoot.com.*

Joanna Slan is the Business Storyteller, known for her inspirational stories in print and on the platform. In addition to speaking full time and teaching salespeople, CEOs, teachers and presenters to tell stories, Joanna is the author of *Using Stories and Humor: Grab Your Audience* and *I'm Too Blessed to Be Depressed.* For more information or to book her for your next meeting, call toll-free 888-BLESSED (253-7733).

Winona Smith is a wife, mother and church secretary who loves to write. She has contributed to *Devotions for Kids, God's Abundance: 365 Days to a Simpler Life, Shining Star Magazine* and *Keys for Kids,* to mention a few. You may contact her at 9060 Roundtree Dr., Baton Rouge, LA 70818.

Lizanne Southgate and her five children live in Oregon. She is the author of *Mother Musing: Essays and Mental Flossings* and *The Unlikely Princess* (a children's book on finding one's own path). Both are available by writing to P.O. Box 878, Brownsville, OR 97327, or by e-mailing her at *lizannes@proaxis.com.*

Carolyn S. Steele lives in Salt Lake City, Utah, with her husband and four children. Her writing and photography have appeared in various newspapers and magazines, including *Outdoor Photographer, The Family Handyman* and *Old House Interiors.* She also writes historic novels, children's books and technical manuals. When not writing, she enjoys photographing weddings, historic architecture and nature. You may write to her at 9158 Winter Wren Dr., Sandy, UT 84093.

Aline Stomfay-Stitz is an associate professor of education at the University of North Florida, Jacksonville, and a graduate of Barnard College, Case Western Reserve and Northern Illinois University. She is a recognized researcher and author on the topics of peace education, conflict resolution and violence prevention, with a mission to bring about more peaceful classrooms and schools. She can be contacted online at *astomfay@unf.edu.*

Mother Teresa, who died in 1997, became known to the world for her selfless work with the "poorest of the poor" in Calcutta, India. With centers around the world, her Missionaries of Charity continue to help the dying and destitute. To order *No Greater Love*, call New World Library at 800-972-6657 extension 52.

LeAnn Thieman is an author and nationally acclaimed speaker. A member of the National Speakers Association, LeAnn inspires audiences to truly live their priorities and balance their lives physically, mentally and spiritually while making a difference in the world. She coauthored *This Must Be My Brother*, a book recounting her role in the daring rescue of 300 babies during the Vietnam Orphan airlift. To inquire about her books, tapes and presentations, contact her at 112 North College, Fort Collins, CO 80524, by calling toll-free 877-THIEMAN, or by e-mail at *www.LeAnnThieman.com.*

Andrew Toos has contributed cartoons to *Good Housekeeping, Saturday Evening Post, The Washington Post, TV Guide, Omni, McCall's, Readers' Digest* and other periodicals. Andrew created the feature strip Bonnie & Hyde and Loon Mountain which are published in *Journal America, Northwest Comic News, Funny Times* and other periodicals. He has moved into the area of interactive television through his work with the cable station, GTE Mainstreet. His work has also been licensed by the T/Maker Company, one of the largest software clip art companies in the world. To find Andrew's cartoons log on AOL and go to Keyword: Howdy. He can be reached at 860-350-3718 or by fax at 860-355-5137 or by e-mail at *drewtoos@aol.com.*

Colleen Trefz has found that her life's richest blessing has been watching her daughters Amber-Lea, Carli, Chelsea, and son, Elisha grow deep and not just tall. She lives in the Northwest with her husband, Delwyne, her children, a horse, a llama, calves, a pig, four dogs, two cats and a bird. She finds much enjoyment in working in the middle school as a community resource director. She believes that virtues are God's gift to us all and how we develop them and acknowledge them in others is our gift to God. Virtuous Reality is her homegrown program created to enrich peoples' lives by focusing on the most important aspect—who we are not what we do! She is available for inspirational and motivational speaking and character education through creativity. You may reach her at 509-766-7291.

Carole Garbuny Vogel of Lexington, Massachusetts, is a writer and lecturer who specializes in inspirational stories for adults and nonfiction for kids. Known as the "Queen of Natural Disaster," she has authored fifteen books including *Shock Waves Through Los Angeles: The Northridge Earthquake* and *The Great Midwest Flood*. Her book, *Will I Get Breast Cancer? A Q & A for Teenage Girls*, won the Joan Fassler Memorial Book Award for excellence in medical writing. Reach her at: 781-861-0440 or e-mail: *cvogel@world.std.com.*

Jim Willoughby is a cartoonist, author and sculptor living in Prescott, Arizona, with his museum-director wife, Sue, a bossy cat and three dogs. He has authored and illustrated seven books, draws cartoons and writes articles for *Arizona Highways, Southwest Art, Phoenix* magazine and others.

Cara Wilson is an internationally acclaimed speaker, with a magical ability to move an audience to laughter and tears in nano-seconds. Her intense love for and belief in young people enables her to connect to teenagers and adults alike, passing the torch of hope that was given to her by the father of Anne Frank. Also a full-time writer/marketing communicator, Cara is presently working on a wide variety of projects, including another book. She may be reached at Creative Impact Marketing 1838 Westcliff Dr., Ste. 4, Newport Beach, CA 92660 phone: 949-650-0300 fax: 949-650-0337 e-mail: *creativeimpact@msn.com.*

E. Lynne Wright is a freelance writer from Vero Beach, Florida. Her fiction, nonfiction articles, essays and book reviews have been published in the *Cleveland Plain Dealer,* the *Hartford Courant, Woman's Household,* the *Vero Beach Press Journal, Yesterday's Magazette* and numerous literary magazines.

Also available from Vermilion

Chicken Soup for the Soul

Stories may be *the* most powerful teaching tool available to us, especially when the subjects being taught are love, respect and values. In this book the authors share a collected wisdom on love, parenting, heroism, death and the overcoming of obstacles.

Price: £8.99   ISBN: 9780091819569

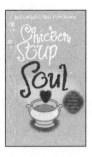

Chicken Soup for the Mother's Soul

This book pays tribute to motherhood – the vocation that requires the skills of a master mediator, mentor, cook, chauffeur and counsellor. These heartwarming stories celebrate the defining moments of motherhood - from birth to letting go as your children leave the nest.

Price: £8.99   ISBN: 9780091819767

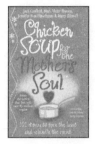

Chicken Soup for the Teenage Soul

Including important lessons on the nature of friendship and love, the value of respect for yourself and others, and dealing with tough issues like death, suicide and the loss of love, this is your handbook for surviving and succeeding during these exciting but sometimes difficult years.

Price: £8.99   ISBN: 9780091826406

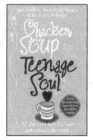

Order these titles direct from www.rbooks.co.uk/chickensoup

Also available from Vermilion

Chicken Soup for the Woman's Soul

This tender collection of stories honours the strength and reveals and the beauty of women's spirits. Whether you're a career woman or stay-at-home mother, teenager or young woman just starting out in the world, this delightful book will be a treasured companion for years to come.

Price: £8.99   ISBN: 9780091825065

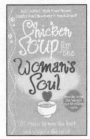

Chicken Soup for the New Mother's Soul

Read about the unique love, the unbreakable bond and the unforgettable moments between mother and child in these heartwarming tales and gain courage and strength in knowing that you too are a wonderful mother.

Price: £8.99   ISBN: 9780091923501

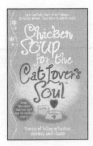

Chicken Soup for the Cat Lover's Soul

Cats have been our treasured companions and soulmates for many years. This touching collection of stories celebrates the special bond we share with

chickensoup